AI

Foods to Promote and Support

Health and Healing

Eat to feel and look great!

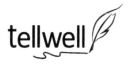

Tellwell Talent

www.tellwell.ca

ISBN

978-1-7730-2877-4 (Paperback)

978-0-2288-4948-3 (eBook)

CONTENTS

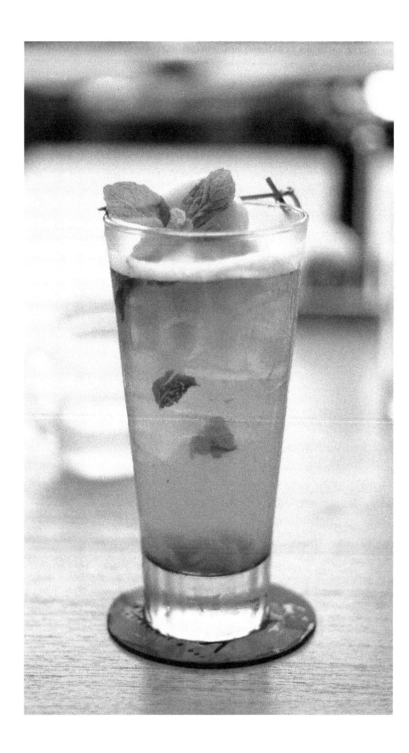

ACKNOWLEDGEMENTS

I would like to thank my friends and family for assisting me in trying out different foods for better health and for encouraging me in the preparation of this work.

Thank you to my Nutrition Instructor at Elevated Learning Academy, Meg Oechslin for her support, assistance and encouragement in putting together this book.

Special thanks to my spiritual parents, Professor E.H. Guti and his wife, Doctor Eunor Guti for the encouragement to work "Talents" - making use of our God-given gifts to bless others and ourselves. That surely inspired me to write the book.

I was also motivated to research on ways for relief from different ailments and problems after talking to friends and fellow church members who agreed to try out some of the foods mentioned. They reported back how they were helped and so to them, I also extend my gratitude for sharing and agreeing to try the foods out. Most images in this book are credited to Unsplash.com

DISCLAIMER

My aim in this book is to provide an easy reference to some information about foods and diseases - tips on prevention and control of some common diseases, illnesses and other health problems based on my own experience and that of others, including close friends and relatives. The contents of the book are not intended to offer personal medical advice. One should seek the advice of a physician or other qualified health provider with any questions one may have regarding a medical condition. Never disregard professional medical advice or delay in seeking it because of something you have read in this book.

The good thing about the foods mentioned is that these are natural methods of healing and preventing involving foods that one needs to eat anyway. Also, remember, these foods are mostly for prevention or for treatment or easing mild symptoms of diseases or other health problems.

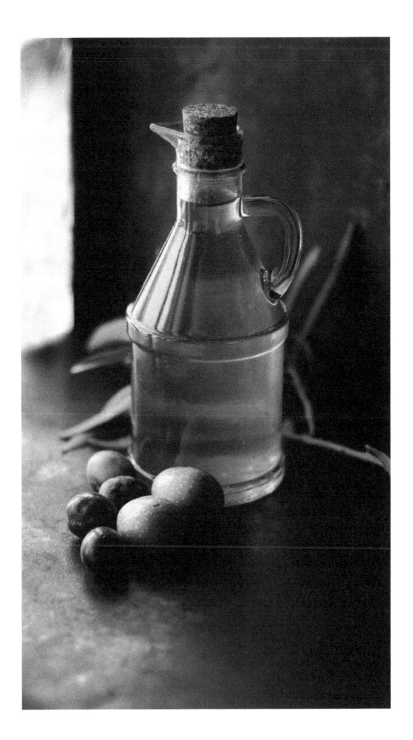

FOREWORD

I first met Anna Maria at Elevated Learning Academy in Edmonton summer of 2016. She had enrolled as a student in the Applied Nutrition Science Diploma Program, and I had the privilege of serving as her Instructor. Anna Maria was thirsty for knowledge and came seeking a greater understanding of how food impacts health and contributes to healing.

Her keen desire to learn and share her life experience was evident and inspiring. Her personal and profound discovery that select foods can improve specific health conditions was a revelation that initiated her exploration into the field of nutrition.

Anna Maria is passionate about the role of nutrition and power of food in our lives. She is on a mission to share the benefits of wholesome, nutritious food with all who cross her path, both personally and globally. As a pastor, Anna Maria embraces a holistic understanding of nutrition beyond the benefits to the body alone. Nourishment of body, mind and spirit is the ultimate message and undercurrent woven between the lines and pages of this enlightening book.

The power of food in our lives cannot be underestimated. As Hippocrates, the Father of Medicine declared millenniums ago, "Let Food be Thy Medicine, and Medicine Thy Food." Thank you, Anna Maria, for continuing to spread this ancient wisdom and valuable message. By doing so, you are investing in and contributing to the wellness and healing of the world.

With Gratitude,
Meg Oechslin, MSc, RD
Registered Dietitian
Nutrition Coach and Instructor
Edmonton, Alberta

INTRODUCTION

Food as medicine has been known since Biblical times. In the mid-1700s, a Scottish surgeon named James Lind learned that some unknown substance in limes prevented scurvy in British sailors[1]

My Journey to Better Health

I got the idea of writing about this after I had been eating carelessly and not minding how my health was impacted by my diet and lifestyle in general. I naively thought that because of my strong faith in God, He would just miraculously heal me if I fell ill. God, in His mercies, has led me to wisdom on eating right to avoid certain ailments, especially as I age. I was diagnosed with very high Blood Pressure by a Nurse at Bible School about six years ago. She advised me to go see a Doctor and most probably get prescription since the level of my Blood Pressure was too high. I told her that I was going to pray for healing and

---

1   "Foods that fight disease" by Leslie Beck RD, Penguin Canada

God was going to heal me. In the meantime, I kept eating foods laden with salts, fats and sugars. I prayed and since there are no symptoms for High Blood Pressure, I forgot about it and just believed that God would take care of my High Blood Pressure and I did very little to lower it.

A year later, I decided to check myself at a Pharmacy and I realized that my Blood Pressure was still very high. That is when I thought of researching on what I should do to lower my Blood Pressure naturally and I found out about foods that I could eat. Of those foods, I just took a handful of **blueberries** a day for 4 days. I went back to check and my Blood Pressure had gone down to normal. That was when I realized how our diet can be so crucial to our health. I then began to investigate the power of different foods for different illnesses.

Another incident that led me to investigate foods and diseases was when one day I realized that I could not see clearly to read the print in my Bible which I had been using for a long time. I then did some research on the foods to eat to improve my eyesight. I incorporated more foods with vitamin A like **carrots, bell peppers, cantaloupes, pumpkins and sweet potatoes** and after some time my eyesight improved.

I have therefore compiled a list of some key foods that help to prevent and to lessen the effects of different ailments. I have compiled the list in alphabetical order of ailments for easy reference. The pictures on each ailment page are also for easy and quick reference and I use pictures of my favorites.

Sometimes when I feel that my diet does not have enough of the vitamins I need, I use supplements. This list is just to help. It is not exhaustive, and one is not limited to it. In most cases, the foods work gradually. So one needs to be patient.

I have presented most foods without suggestions of how to prepare them for consumption, assuming that most people who will refer to the book have some idea of how best to prepare them. Most of the foods can be eaten raw, e.g. the fruits and vegetables in salads or smoothies or freshly squeezed juices.

Also remember, eating the right foods alone is not enough for good health. One needs to do other things like drinking plenty of water, exercising, sleeping well and avoiding stressful situations.

In this second edition, I have included a lot of tropical foods which are readily available and not so expensive, for example, okra, pumpkin leaves and lemon and orange peels. I have also dedicated the second last page to some of the superfoods easily found in Tropical countries, especially in Southern Africa.

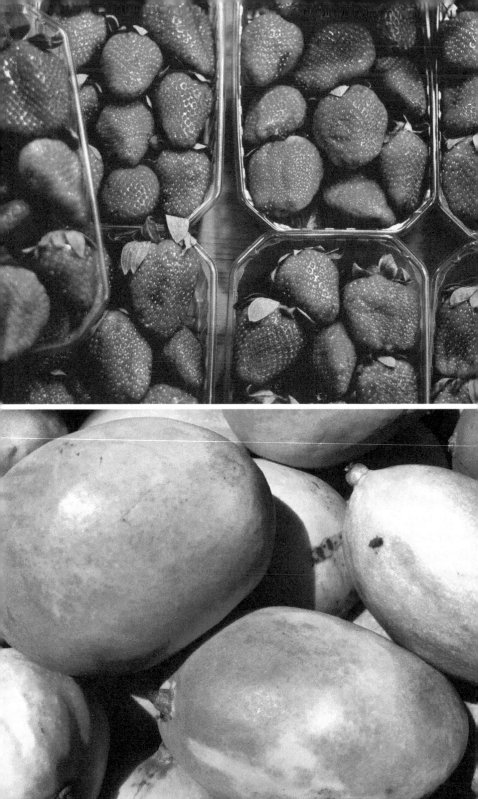

ACNE

Foods to Nourish Skin or for a Smoother Skin

Foods to Eat[2]

- Foods with **omega-3 fatty acids.** This includes **salmon, flax seeds, and walnuts.**

- **Antioxidant rich foods.** Antioxidant foods are not only good for your health, but they also give your skin an extra dose of goodness. Antioxidant rich foods like **cherries, berries, green tea and spinach** attack free radicals in your body that cause skin damage and breakouts.

- **Foods rich in selenium: Brazil nuts, almonds, onion, garlic, and whole grains** are all sources of selenium, which is also a powerful antioxidant.

---

2   "Foods that fight disease" by Leslie Beck RD, Penguin Canada

These foods help preserve your skin's elasticity and reduce inflammation.

- Foods **rich in zinc**: Most **Nuts, whole grains** and **legumes**[3]

- Foods **rich in vitamin C**: **Melons, oranges, tomatoes, and strawberries** all boost your immune system and strengthen your cell walls. These foods will help protect your skin from acne scarring and activate healing powers to amend damaged or irritated skin.

- Foods **rich in vitamin E.** This includes **nuts, soybeans, almonds, leafy greens and eggs.** Vitamin E rich foods also help protect your skin from scarring. An easy way of getting Vitamin E is by using **Olive Oil** in cooking and in salads.

- **Foods with high water conten**t. This means **drink plenty of water.** Keeping your body hydrated is one of the best things you can do for yourself and for your skin. In addition to drinking 1/2 your body weight in ounces throughout the day, eating foods with a high water content like **watermelon** and **cucumbers**, and also **parsley** will free your system of toxins as well.

- **Foods rich in vitamin A.** Foods that give your body vitamin A are rich in beta-carotene, which enhances the benefits of selenium - the powerful antioxidant

3   IBID

mentioned above. Include **carrots, bell peppers, cantaloupes, and sweet potatoes** into your daily diet.

- **Foods high in magnesium.** These foods are awesome acne fighters because magnesium helps to balance out acne-inducing hormones. Try munching on **artichokes, oatmeal, brown rice, and figs** to get hormonal acne under control.

Tropical Foods

- **Mangoes** are also high in water content and can be used as a skin cleanser: Mangoes help you unclog your pores and add freshness to the face. Mangoes are applicable to any skin type. They help clear clogged pores that cause acne. Just slice a mango into thin pieces and keep them on your face for 10 to 15 minutes and then wash your face and see the results.[4]

- **Lemon Peels.** They help in preventing and fighting skin problems such as wrinkles, acne, pigmentation and dark spots. This is due to the free radicles in them. They are also rich in antioxidants which tend to detoxify the skin to a very great extent.

---

4   https://healthimpactnews.
    com/2013/17-reasons-why-you-need-a-mango-every-day/

- **Orange Peels.** They help cure multiple skin problems such as blackheads, dead cells, acne, pores, dark circles and dry skin. It also helps brighten your skin.

- The peels can be boiled in water and drank as tea. Peel one orange or one lemon and boil the peels in 2 cups of water for 2 mins and drink as tea daily. They make delicious tea and you can boil them separately or together.

- **Pumpkin Leaves.** Due to the presence of anti-oxidants in abundance, these leaves are known to slow down the ageing process.

- **Okra.** The high vitamin C content helps the growth and rejuvenation of skin cells and collagen, which keeps skin looking smoother, younger and healthier

Foods to Avoid

Some foods seem to be associated with skin damage. For example, some research suggests **that a diet high in processed or refined carbohydrates and unhealthy fats promotes skin aging.**[5]

Refined foods like white **bread**, white **rice**, white **refined flour**, **French fries**, and **mashed potatoes** are some of the worst things to have in your diet if you want flawless skin. **Refined sugar** is to be avoided because it makes your

---

5   http://www.mayoclinic.org/healthy-lifestyle/adult-health/
    expert-answers/healthy-skin

blood sugar levels spike, which then causes acne outbreaks. **High Sodium foods** are foods packed with salt which not only make your body bloat up, they also cause problems to your skin. To avoid pimples from flaring up, try to limit the amount of processed or prepared foods in your diet. **Substitute canned or frozen vegetables with fresh ones.**[6]

These foods to be avoided are not only for acne but for overall health.

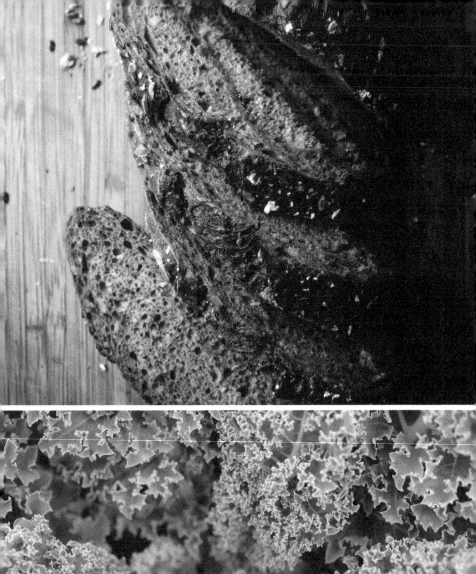
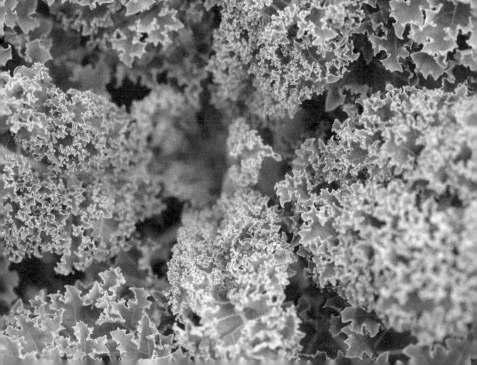

ALCOHOLISM

Foods that Support Recovery and Reduce Craving for Alcohol

An alcoholic is defined as a person who follows a regular pattern of alcohol consumption (daily, weekly, or binge drinking), needs alcohol to function adequately (psychological dependence), or has developed a physical tolerance and/or physical distress with withdrawal. Alcoholism affects almost all the organs of the body, but particularly the liver, which contains the enzymes needed for alcohol metabolism[7]

---

[7] http://www.consultant360.com/n411/articles/
alcohol-abuse-and-nutrition

It is important for alcoholics to avoid **refined sugars** and **caffeine**, as they stress blood sugar control mechanisms and may increase the craving for alcohol.[8]

The key, addiction experts say, is to choose foods that do one of three things: Improve digestion, promote steady blood sugar throughout the day or support brain chemistry.

There are good reasons these factors help manage sobriety. Healthy digestion optimizes the absorption of amino acids, vitamins and minerals that reduce cravings for alcohol. Having steady blood sugar all day normalizes insulin and leptin, hormones responsible for regulating hunger. And getting enough **lean protein** ensures optimal levels of neurotransmitters associated with reward and feelings of well-being. No one food will cure cravings for alcohol. Rather, to work, craving-busting foods must be part of a balanced diet that includes **complex carbohydrates, lean protein, healthy fat and fiber.** Here are some of the alcohol craving busters from addiction experts:[9]

- **100% whole-grain bread.** Because alcohol is converted to sugar in the body, when you stop drinking, your body still craves the sugar. So you drink more alcohol because of the sugar craving which therefore equates to alcohol craving. The complex

---

8   Michael Murray N.D. Et al, "The Encyclopedia of Healing Foods", Atria Books, New York, NY 10020 2005

9   Ibid

carbohydrates in whole-grain bread metabolize slowly and kill sugar cravings for longer. Whole grains also provide a lot of nutritional value as they contain **protein, unsaturated fats, vitamins and minerals.** Look for whole-grain bread with no added sugar. Also: **brown rice, quinoa, oats** and **barley**

- **Raw spinach. Spinach and parsley** provide vitamins, minerals and fiber, and they help regulate metabolism. They also contain L-glutamine, an amino acid that decreases anxiety and reduces cravings. Spinach and parsley should be eaten raw, as L-glutamine breaks down during the cooking process. Also, raw parsley

- **Peanut butter.** Peanut butter and Brazil nuts are good sources of dietary fiber, vitamin B and protein, which contain amino acids that are essential for the production of dopamine, a key neurotransmitter associated with mood and the feeling of well-being. Other excellent sources of protein include **beans, tofu, dairy products and Brazil nuts.**

- **Salmon, tuna and mackerel** are loaded with protein and **vitamin D**, which has been shown to decrease depression and stabilize mood. Coldwater fish such as salmon and mackerel are also full of healthy polyunsaturated fats and are among the best sources of **omega-3 fatty acids**, which have been shown to decrease depression, regulate mood and improve cognitive function — all of which could work to reduce cravings.

- **Liver** and other foods that contain **Vitamin D**, such as **fish, eggs dark leafy greens, milk (fortified with the Vitamin D) cow, soy and almond.**

- **Bananas.** Heavy alcohol consumption causes short-term euphoria, but over time it reduces levels of the mood-boosting brain chemical dopamine. Reduction in dopamine can cause cravings. **Bananas and sunflower seeds** raise dopamine levels naturally. In addition, the B vitamins in bananas increase serotonin levels, another neurotransmitter that reduces depression and anxiety.

- **Peas and Leafy Greens** -The **B vitamins** in these foods are extremely important in alcohol recovery and craving reduction, according to the University of Maryland Medical Center. This group of vitamins provides your body with energy to combat fatigue, helps in the production of red blood cells for proper brain and heart functions as well as helps to metabolize nutrients properly during digestion. These vitamins are also important for increasing serotonin production, which helps to lower the incidence of depression and anxiety experienced during the initial withdrawal from alcohol. Eating five to eight servings of **fruits and vegetables** daily provides adequate amounts of B vitamins. Choose snacks with **bananas and raisins**, or eat a lunch salad full of greens such as **romaine lettuce, broccoli and spinach**. **Add peas or beets** as a side dish for dinner and enjoy **oranges, grapefruit or melons** for dessert.[10]

· **Walnuts.** Walnuts are loaded with protein and omega-3 fatty acids. Many seeds are also excellent sources of fiber and antioxidants - **flax seeds and chia seeds.**

Mindful Eating and Other Hints

Besides focusing on individual foods, you can adopt eating strategies that reduce cravings. An example is "mindful eating," which simply means slowing down and eating regularly.

Meals should be within four to five hours, and snacks can be fit in between. So, one should be eating every two to three hours. Any type of extreme — such as skipping meals, cutting food groups or eating rapidly — can result in low blood glucose levels, which mimic alcohol cravings.[11]

For the best all-around snack to reduce cravings try a few ounces of **frozen fruit**, a couple of **Brazil nuts**, a

---

10 http://www.livestrong.com/
    article/314904-foods-that-reduce-alcohol-cravings/

11 Ibd

few squares of **dark chocolate**, and a few ounces of **coconut water.**

In fact, research shows that getting plenty of **exercise** increases levels of the hormone leptin — an appetite suppressor — and reduces levels of ghrelin — which creates the sensation of hunger. So, after doing everything right in your diet, exercise as well.

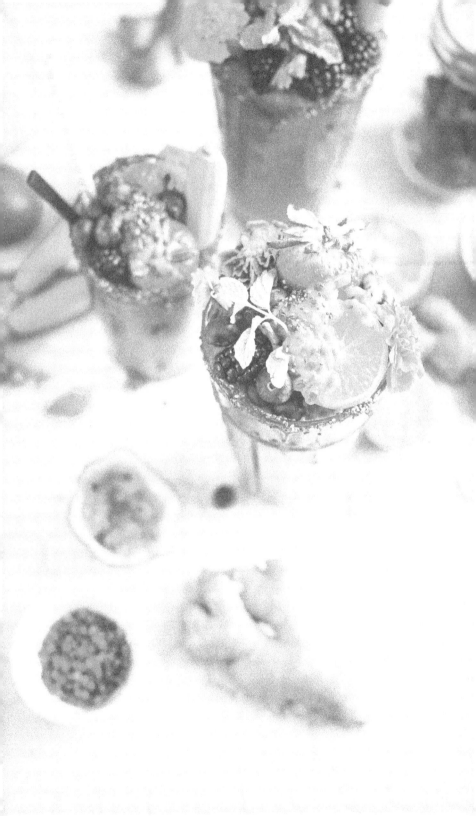

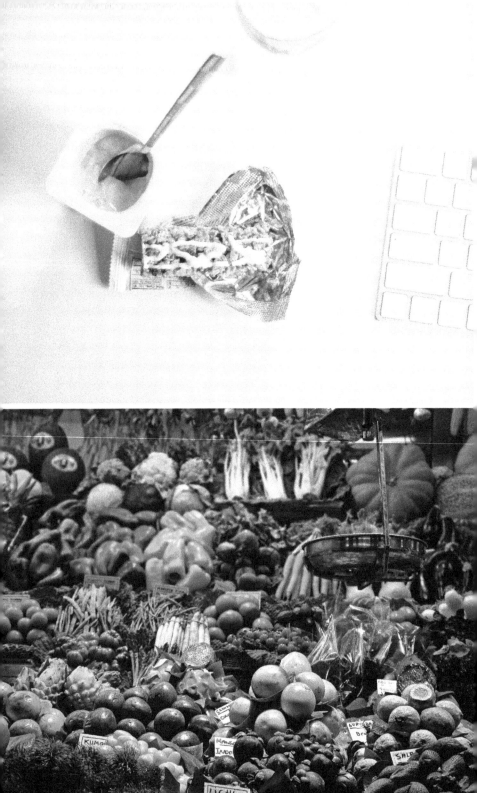

ALLERGY & ASTHMA
Symptom Relievers

- **Green Tea** -Tea contains natural antihistamines which make it a great addition to the diet to reduce allergy symptoms. Histamine is a chemical that the body releases during allergic reactions.

- **Mediterranean Diet** - There is some research to support the idea that adhering to a Mediterranean diet increases a person's chance of controlling their asthma[12]. This diet includes **lots of fruits, vegetables, beans, whole grains, fish, and olive oil, with a lesser amount of meat.**

- **Yogurt and Other Probiotics** - Add yogurt and other sources of probiotics to your diet. Probiotics, which you can get from **yogurt, miso, fermented milk,**

12   http://www.everydayhealth.com/allergy-photos/allergies-and-food.aspx#08

and dietary supplements, can help regulate your immune system so you'll have fewer allergy symptoms.

- **Go Low-Cal and Lose Weight** - Researchers have found that being obese may worsen asthma.[13]

- **Low-Salt Diet** - Studies have found that eating a diet higher in salt may be associated with more severe asthma, and small studies have found that eating a low-salt diet can improve lung function, decrease symptoms, and reduce the need for medications in people with asthma. Good ways to reduce salt in your diet include eating **plenty of fresh vegetables** and cutting down on processed foods like frozen dinners and canned soups.[14]

- **Omega-3 Intake** - Some research indicates that eating a diet rich in **omega-3 fatty acids** may be helpful for reducing asthma symptoms. You can get more omega-3s in your diet by eating **fatty fish such as salmon, herring, sardines, mackerel, and albacore tuna.**

- **Avoid Fast Food** - A New Zealand study of more than 1,300 kids found that those who ate hamburgers occasionally or at least once a week were more likely to have asthma symptoms than kids who never ate burgers. A diet designed to reduce asthma and allergy symptoms with foods like **fruits, vegetables** and **fish** might not leave a lot of room for fast food.[15]

---

13 Ibd

14 Ibd

15 http everydayhealth.com/diet-nutrition/101/nutrition-basics.

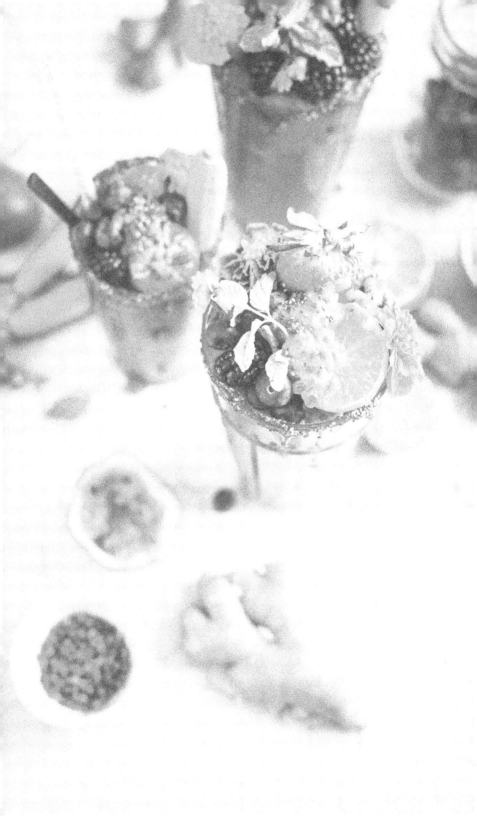

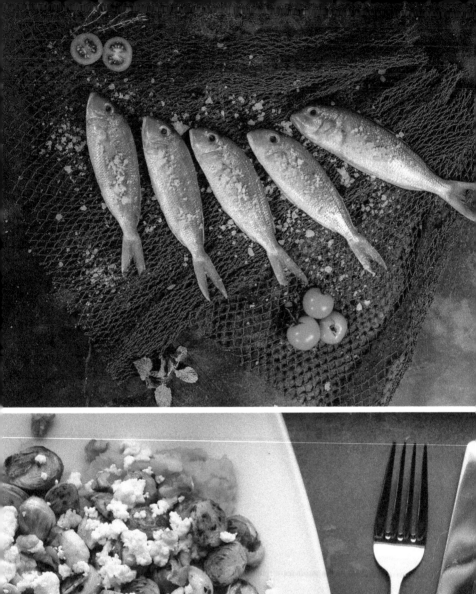
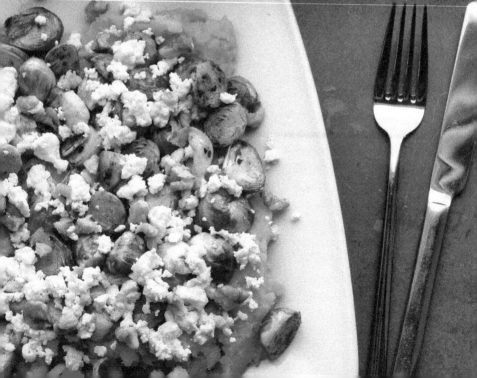

ALZHEIMER'S

Foods that Nourish the Brain or Improve Memory

Salmon and other cold-water fish, such as halibut, tuna, mackerel and sardines, which are rich in omega-3 fatty acids. Other omega-3 sources include beans, some nuts, flax seeds and healthy oils, like olive oil.

Berries and dark-skinned fruits which are rich in antioxidants. Some of the fruits that pack the most punch are blueberries, blackberries, strawberries, raspberries, plums, oranges, red grapes and cherries.

· **Foods and Beverages High in Flavonoids**

Plants have created an arsenal of protective chemicals called polyphenols to defend themselves against predators such as herbivores. Flavonoids are among the toughest of these, and they also fall into the antioxidant category.

Flavonoid-rich fruits include **apples, blueberries, cranberries, and grapefruit. Vegetables with flavonoids include asparagus, Brussels sprouts, cabbage, garlic, kale, kohlrabi, kidney and lima beans, onions, peas, and spinach.** One study found that people who drank fruit and **vegetable juices such as orange, apple, or tomato** three times a week were less likely to develop Alzheimer's disease.

- **Foods High in Folate**

Doctors have known for years that deficiency of certain B vitamins, particularly folate, can make it difficult to perform some cognitive tasks. New evidence shows that even slightly low levels can have a similar effect because folate, along with vitamins B6 and B12, helps to keep homocysteine levels in check. This amino acid impairs brain function and can dramatically increase a person's risk of Alzheimer's disease (as well as heart disease). The good news is that folate from foods like **dark leafy greens and dried beans** may slow cognitive decline.[16]

Folic acid, vitamin B12, vitamin D, magnesium, and fish oil may help to preserve brain health[17]

---

16   IBID

17   https://www.helpguide.org/articles/alzheimers-dementia/
     alzheimers-and-dementia-prevention.htm

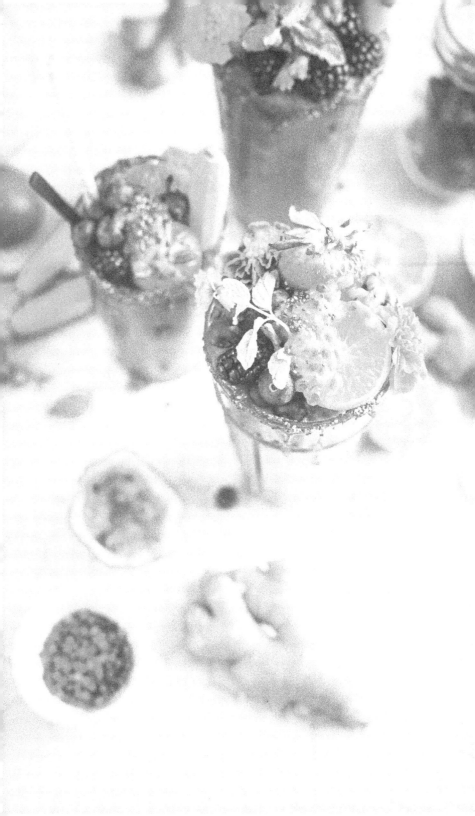

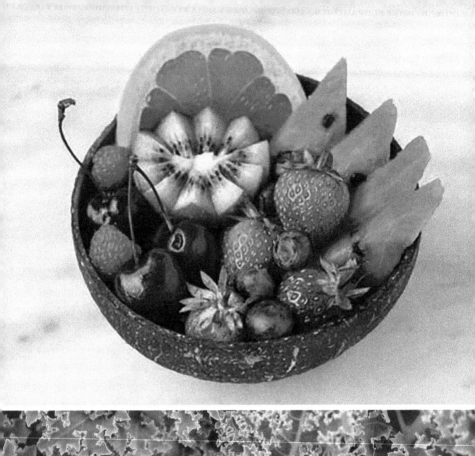

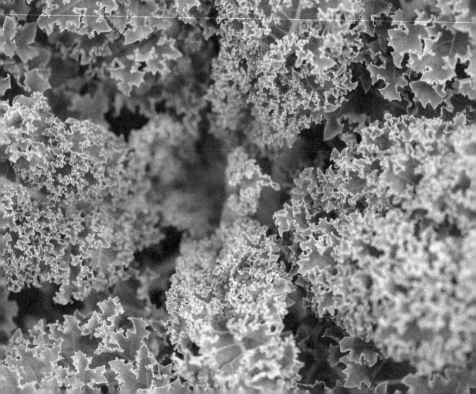

ANEMIA[18]

Foods to Boost Iron Levels

Iron deficiency anemia can be reduced by choosing iron-rich foods.

Foods rich in iron

- **Red meat**
- **Pork**
- **Poultry**
- **Seafood**
- **Legumes, including lentils**
- **Dark green leafy vegetables, such as spinach**
- **Dried fruit, such as raisins and apricots**

---

18   "Foods that fight disease" by Leslie Beck RD, Penguin Canada

- **Iron-fortified cereals, breads and pastas**

- **Peas**

- **Sorghum** - One serving of this rich tropical whole grain contains 47 percent of your daily recommended iron and 55 percent of your phosphorus intake. It's also a good source of magnesium, copper, calcium, zinc and potassium.[19]

The body absorbs more iron from meat than it does from other sources. Those who choose to not eat meat may need to increase their intake of iron-rich, plant-based foods to absorb the same amount of iron as those who eat meat.

- **Foods containing vitamin C enhance iron absorption**

The body's absorption of iron is enhanced by drinking citrus juice or eating other foods rich in **vitamin C** while one eats high-iron foods. **Vitamin C in citrus juices, like orange juice**, helps the body to better absorb dietary iron. **Vitamin C is also found in:**

- **Broccoli**

- **Grapefruit**

- **Kiwi**

- **Leafy greens**

- **Melons**

---

19   http://curetick.com/sorghum-benefits-and-side-effects/

- **Oranges**

- **Peppers**

- **Strawberries**

- **Tangerines**

- **Tomatoes**

- **Mangoes**

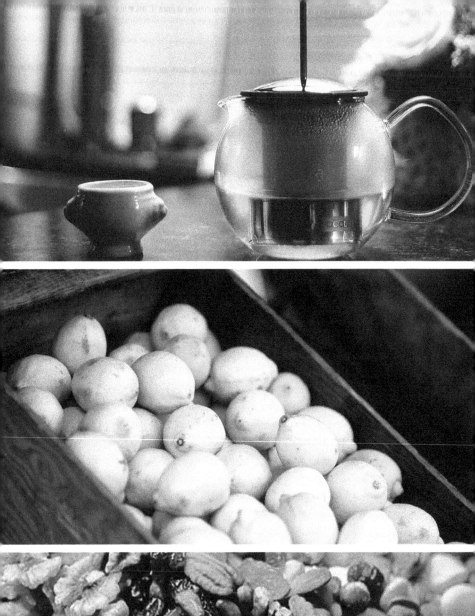
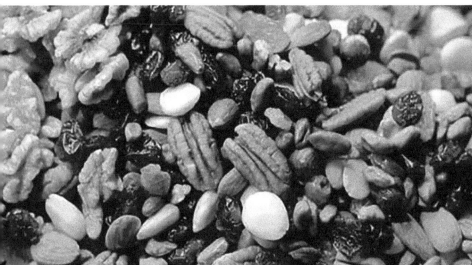

ANXIETY

Foods that Calm Anxiety

- **Chamomile, lemon balm, fish and some types of nuts** can help reduce anxiety levels when consumed regularly.

- Regular consumption of **foods that are high in omega-3 fatty acids** can lower stress hormones and reduce stress. **Nuts, such as walnuts, and fish are common sources of omega-3 fatty acids.** Between 1 and 3 grams of omega-3 fatty acids per day is recommended to reduce anxiety.

- **Fish also contains L-lysine,** an amino acid that may help reduce stress. Foods that contain high levels of **zinc, magnesium and vitamin B-12** are recommended as a deficiency in these vitamins and minerals can result in an increased risk of anxiety. **Almonds and spinach** are good sources of zinc. **Fish** is a good source of vitamin B-12, and **cashews** provide magnesium.

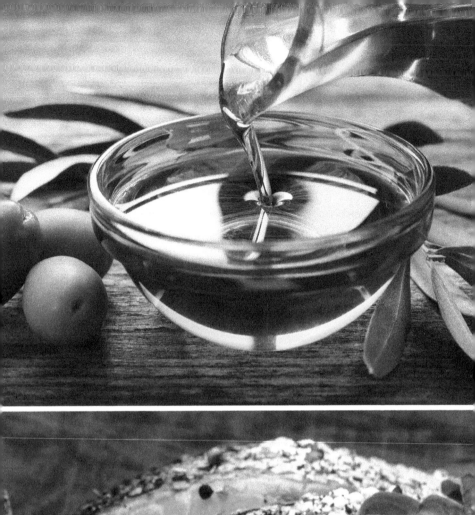
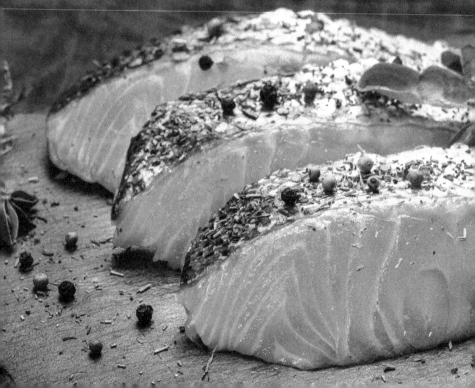

ARTHRITIS
Foods that Relieve Arthritis

- **Fish** is a great source of omega-3 fatty acids. While some foods increase inflammation in the body, omega-3 fatty acids decrease inflammation and suppress the production of enzymes that erode cartilage. Fish is greatly beneficial for people with rheumatoid arthritis.

- **Soy** is another food that has the inflammation-busting benefits of omega-3 fatty acids. **Soybeans, tofu or edamame** are heart-healthy foods that are low in fat, high in protein and fibre, and a great option for vegans and vegetarians.

- **Olive oil** contains heart-healthy monounsaturated fats and oleocanthal, which is a natural phenolic compound that has similar properties to non-steroidal, anti-inflammatory drugs. Oleocanthal lowers the production of enzymes that cause inflammation. Olive oil works well for rheumatoid arthritis and osteoarthritis.

- **Green tea** is rich in polyphenols, which are antioxidants that reduce inflammation and inhibit cartilage destruction.

- **Dairy** - Consuming low-fat dairy products such as **milk, yoghurt and cheese** increases bone strength as these foods are rich in both calcium and Vitamin D.[20]

---

20 Vitamin D is vital for calcium absorption, and it is known to boost the immune system. If you're vegan or lactose intolerant, you can reach for dairy-free sources of calcium and Vitamin D such as leafy green vegetables

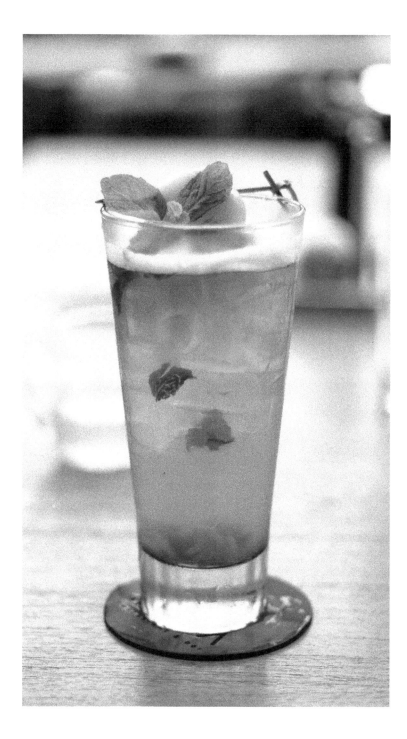

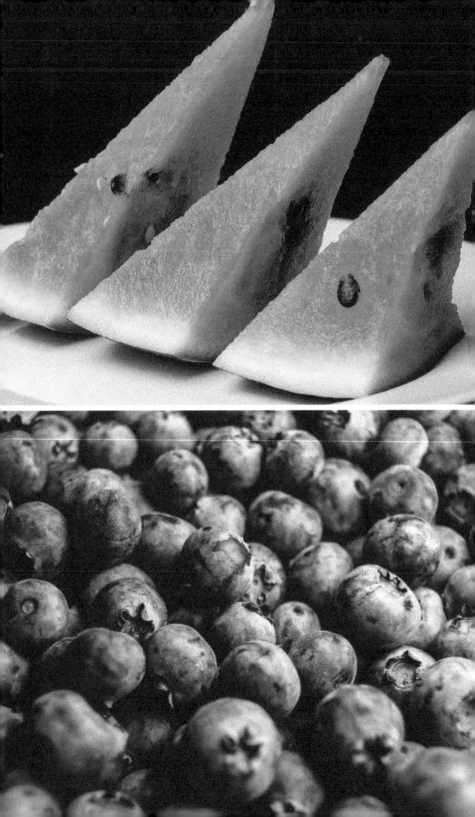

BLOOD PRESSURE
Foods to Lower Blood Pressure

- **Blueberries** - Just eating one cup of blueberries or strawberries a week may help you lower your risk of high blood pressure.[21] Eating more darker-colored foods that contain compounds called anthocyanins — may cut your risk of developing it.

- **Anthocyanins** — found mainly in **fruits and vegetables** such as **blueberries, raspberries, strawberries, cranberries, black currants, eggplants and blood oranges** — seem to protect against high blood pressure.

- **Cereal** - Having a bowl of breakfast cereal, especially whole-grain, high-fiber cereals like **oatmeal, oat squares, bran flakes or shredded wheat,** can reduce your chance of developing high blood pressure, Harvard

---

21   Joan Rattner Heilman. AARP Bulletin. March 8, 2011

University researchers recently found. The more servings of cereal you eat a week, the greater the benefits. One can double their health rewards by topping their cereal with berries.[22] One should also avoid the sweet refined cereals. They do more harm than good.

- **Potato** - A baked potato is high in potassium and magnesium - two important minerals that can help fight high blood pressure.

- **Halibut, spinach, bananas, soybeans, kidney beans and plain non-fat yogurt** are also high in potassium and magnesium

- **Beet** - Drinking a glass of **beet juice** can lower blood pressure within just a few hours because of the nitrate in them. Other nitrate-rich foods include **spinach, lettuce, cabbage, carrots** and **whole beets**

- **Skim milk** - Drinking low-fat milk makes women less likely to develop high blood pressure. In other words, low-fat dairy products can reduce a woman's risk of developing hypertension.

- **Dark Chocolate** - Flavonoids in chocolate help to lower blood pressure. Eating one-ounce square of dark chocolate daily can help lower blood pressure, especially in people who already have hypertension.

---

22 Idbd

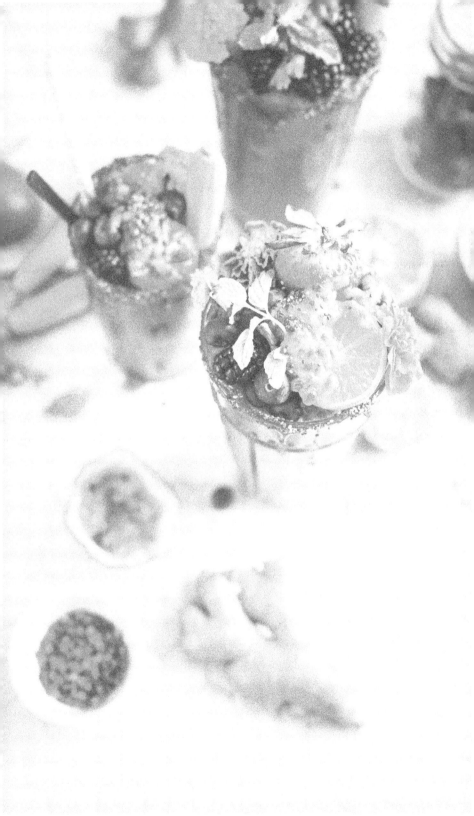

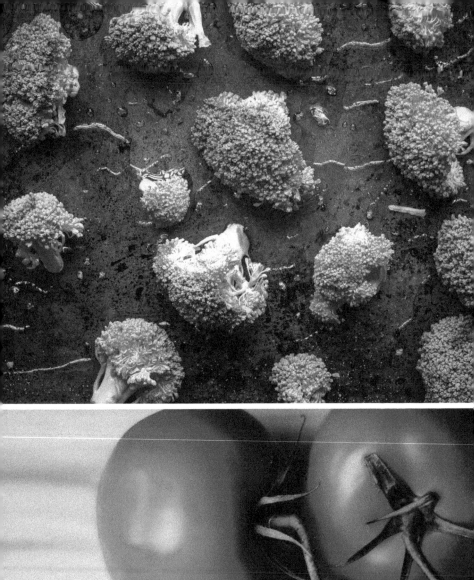
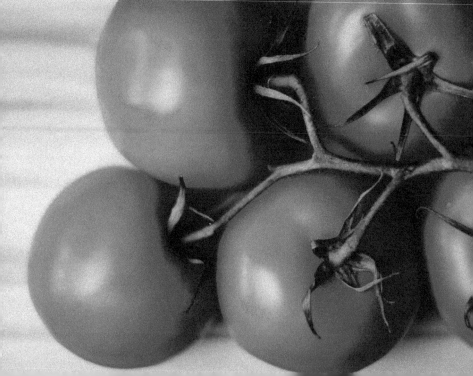

CANCER

Foods to Prevent or Abate Cancer

Aim for five to nine daily servings of all kinds of **fruits and vegetables**, especially the following:

- **Broccoli** - Helps fight: breast, liver, lung, prostate, skin, stomach, and bladder cancers

- **Berries** - All **berries** are packed with cancer-fighting phytonutrients.

- **Tomatoes** - This juicy fruit is the best dietary source of lycopene, a carotenoid that gives tomatoes their red hue. The biggest benefits come from **cooked tomatoes** since the heating process increases the amount of lycopene our bodies are able to absorb.

- **Walnuts** - Help fight: breast and prostate cancers. Having an ounce of walnuts a day may yield the best benefits.

- **Garlic-** helps fight breast, colon, esophageal, and stomach cancers. Crushed garlic is better as crushing helps release beneficial enzymes.

- **Sorghum** - Certain phytochemicals in sorghum have been shown to have cancer-inhibiting properties, particularly in gastrointestinal and skin cancers.

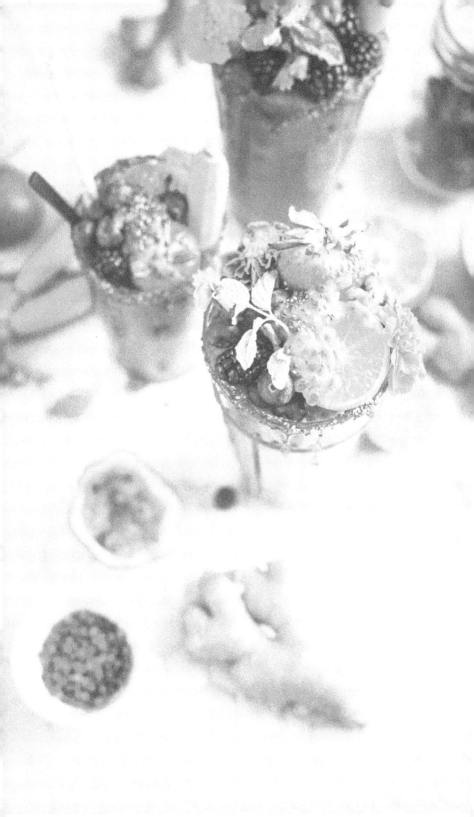

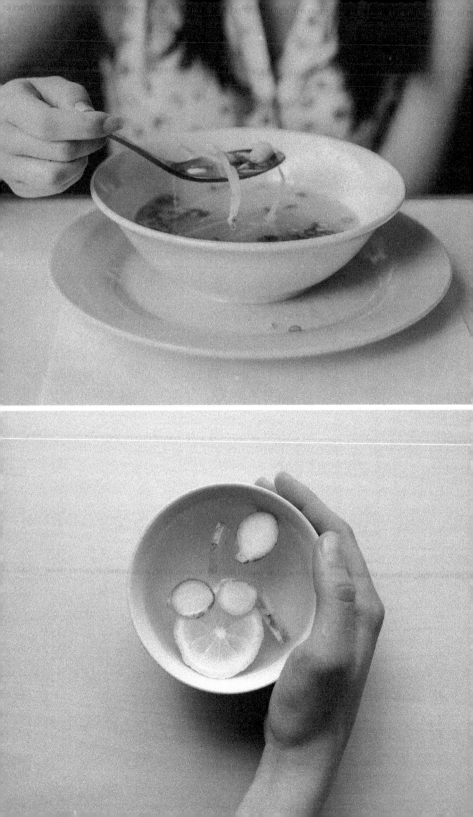

COMMON COLDS

To Nurse the Common Cold

- Gargle with salt water and then have some **chicken soup**.

- Drink **lots of fluids** (such as water and tea). The American Lung Association recommends drinking eight glasses of water or juice per day when trying to get rid of a common cold. Staying hydrated helps moisturize the lining of the nose and throat, which makes mucus easier to clear. Avoid caffeinated or alcoholic drinks, as they can cause dehydration.

- **Garlic**[23]

- **Turmeric**[24]

- **Eat chicken soup.**

---

23 http://www.health.com/health/gallery/

24 http://dailyburn.com/life/health/healthy-tips-natural-flavors.

- Take vitamin C.

- **Ginger**

- **Get plenty of rest**

- **Take a steamy shower or use a humidifier**

- **Vitamin D** - A Japanese study showed that **Vitamin D** is more effective at preventing the flu than a vaccine! The way Vitamin D works is by stimulating your immune system and rallying T cells to start fighting off infections.[25]

---

25 http://www.health.com/health/gallery/

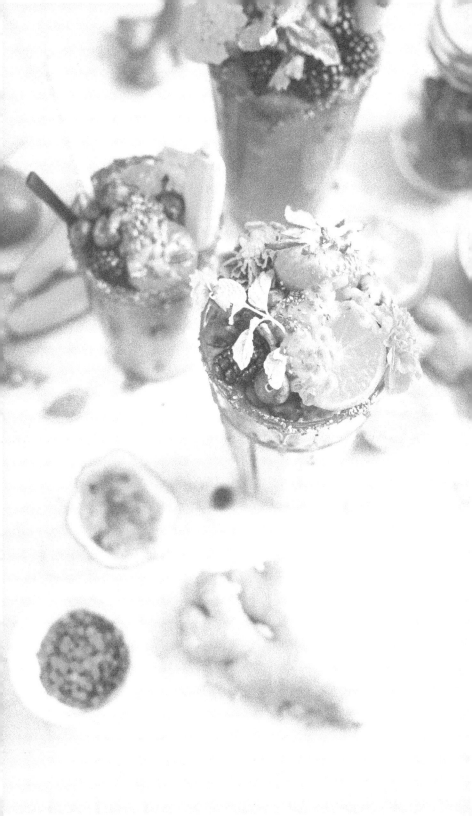

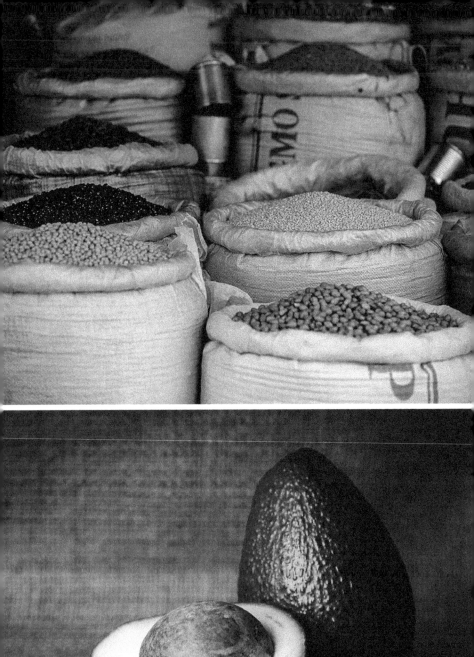
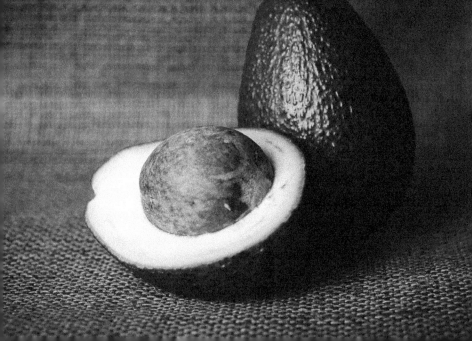

CHOLESTEROL[26]

Foods to Balance or Lower Cholesterol

- **Soy** - Reducing saturated fat is the single most important dietary change one can make to cut blood cholesterol. Used as a replacement for meat and cheese, **soy foods** help your heart by slashing the amount of saturated fat that you eat.

- **Beans** - Except for wheat bran, no food is more fiber-rich than beans. And beans are especially high in cholesterol-lowering soluble fiber. Eating a cup of any type of beans a day—particularly kidney, navy, pinto, black, chickpea, or butter beans—can lower cholesterol by as much as 10% in 6 weeks.

---

26 http://www.prevention.com/food/
    food-remedies/10-best-cholesterol-lowering-foods

- **Salmon** - Research has shown certain types of fat protect against high cholesterol. Omega-3 fatty acids—found in salmon and other cold-water fish—help lower "bad" LDL cholesterol, raise "good" HDL cholesterol, and lower triglycerides. Salmon is an excellent source of protein because it is high in omega-3 fatty acids called EPA and DHA that are good for your heart while low in cholesterol and saturated fat.

- **Avocado** - Avocados are a great source of heart-healthy monounsaturated fat, a type of fat that may help to raise levels of HDL ("good"cholesterol) while lowering levels of LDL ("bad" cholesterol). Beta-sitosterol reduces the amount of cholesterol absorbed from food. So, the combination of beta-sitosterol and monounsaturated fat makes the avocado an excellent cholesterol buster.

- **Garlic** - For thousands of years, garlic has been used in nearly every culture in the world. Its nutritional value and flavor have made it a kitchen staple. Ancient Egyptians ate garlic for stamina. In modern times, garlic has been found to lower cholesterol, prevent blood clots, reduce blood pressure, and protect against infections. Now research has found that it helps stop artery-clogging plaque at its earliest stage called nano plaque. Garlic keeps individual cholesterol particles from sticking to artery walls.[27]

- **Spinach** - Spinach contains lots of lutein, the sunshine-yellow pigment found in dark green leafy vegetables and egg yolks. Lutein already has a "golden" reputation for guarding against age-related macular degeneration, a leading cause of blindness. Now research suggests that just a ½ cup of a lutein-rich food daily also guards against heart attacks by helping artery walls "shrug off" cholesterol invaders that cause clogging.[28]

- **Green Tea** - Tea, iced or hot is rich in antioxidant compounds. Studies prove that tea helps to keep blood vessels relaxed and prevent blood clots. Flavonoids, the major antioxidants in tea, have been shown to prevent the oxidation of LDL cholesterol that leads to plaque formation on artery walls. These powerful antioxidants may reduce cholesterol and even lower blood pressure.

- **Walnuts, Cashews and Almonds** - A moderate-fat diet that is rich in the healthy monounsaturated fats found in nuts may be twice as good for your heart as a low-fat diet. Nuts also have vitamin E, magnesium,

---

27 http://www.prevention.com/health/health-concerns/
how-lower-blood-pressure-naturally

28 IBD

copper, and phytochemicals that have been linked to heart health. And walnuts are also rich in omega-3s. People who eat nuts regularly have less heart disease and other illnesses than people who don't. The heart-healthy monounsaturated fats they contain are also better for your joints than the polyunsaturated fats found in corn and safflower oils.

- **Chocolate** - Choose the dark or bittersweet kind. Compared to milk chocolate, it has more than three times as many antioxidants. These flavonoid antioxidants work to keep blood platelets from sticking together and may even help keep your arteries unclogged. Milk chocolate is good too. Research shows that about an ounce of chocolate a day increases good cholesterol and prevents bad cholesterol from oxidizing.

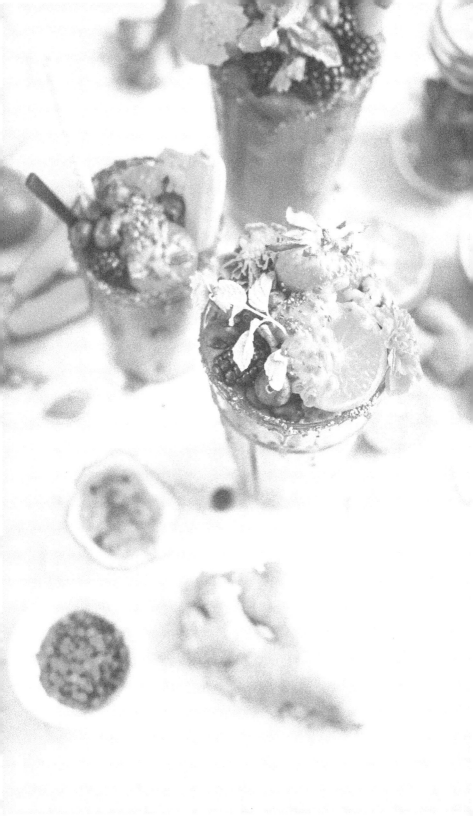

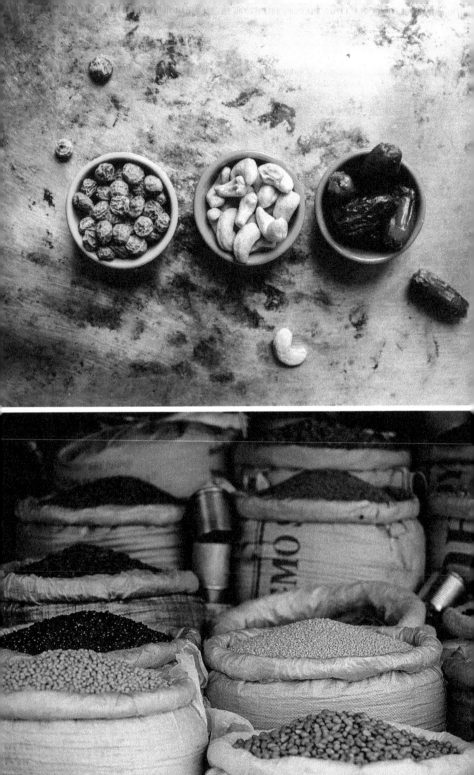

CONSTIPATION
Foods to Counteract Constipation

- **Dried fruit** such as **dates, figs, prunes, apricots,** and **raisins**, are all examples of great sources of dietary fiber that act as a constipation remedy. **Prunes** are great because they not only are high in fiber, but also contain sorbitol, which is a natural laxative[29]

- **Berries** - Eat the following: **raspberries, blackberries, and strawberries.** They all have a good amount of fiber. A half-cup of fresh strawberries provides 2 grams of fiber while the same size serving of blackberries will provide 3.8 grams and raspberries 4 grams. Berries also are low in calories, so you can eat a big bowl of plain berries with low-fat whipped

---

29 http://www.everydayhealth.com/
    digestive-health-pictures/10-foods-that-help-relieve-constipation

cream as dessert or toss them on your breakfast cereal, or mix them in pancakes.[30]

· **Popcorn** - Popcorn is a good source of fibre but adding too much salt and butter could undo some of its benefits. Popcorn is a whole grain, and increasing the whole-grains in your diet is an effective constipation remedy.

· **Beans**[31] - Beans are incredibly versatile and can be tossed into any number of salads, soups, casseroles, and pasta. A half-cup serving of navy beans will provide 9.5 grams of fiber, while a similar size serving of kidney beans provides 8.2 grams.

· **Whole-Grain Bread** - To avoid constipation, eat whole-grain breads. Whole-grain breads are low in fat and high in dietary fiber and complex carbohydrates.

· **High-Fiber Cereal** - Choosing a cereal that has at least 5 grams of fiber per serving is a good start. One can also add fiber to a favorite cereal by sprinkling a tablespoon of wheat bran or flaxseed on top.

· **Broccoli** - Broccoli is a great source of fiber. It is low in calories and a great source of nutrients. Raw

---

30 http://www.everydayhealth.com/digestive-health-pictures/how-to-experiment-with-an-ulcerative-colitis-diet.asp

31 http://www.everydayhealth.com/columns/johannah-sakimura-nutrition-sleuth/learn-love-legumes-benefits-beans/

broccoli is better, since cooking it can reduce its fiber content. If cooked broccoli is preferred, steaming, broiling, or baking is better to avoid extra calories. A small amount of olive oil, salt, and pepper is good for additional flavor.

- **Plums, Pears, and Apples** - Raw fruits can be a constipation remedy because fruit, is high in dietary fiber. Plums, pears, and apples are good choices because much of the fiber can be found in their edible skins. Plums, pears, and apples are also high in pectin, a naturally occurring fiber.

- **Nuts** - Nuts are also full of fiber. Among the best are **Brazil nuts, peanuts, and walnuts**. A 1-ounce serving of almonds provides 3.3 grams of fiber, while a similar size serving of pistachios will provide 2.9 grams of fiber, and pecans 2.7 grams. However, nuts are calorie-dense and therefore one should avoid having too many.

- **Baked Potatoes** - A medium baked potato, with skin, has 3.8 grams of fiber. A baked sweet potato with its skin provides 4.8 grams of fiber. Boiling and mashing potatoes with its skin is another good way to serve them. French fries are high in fat and should be avoided.

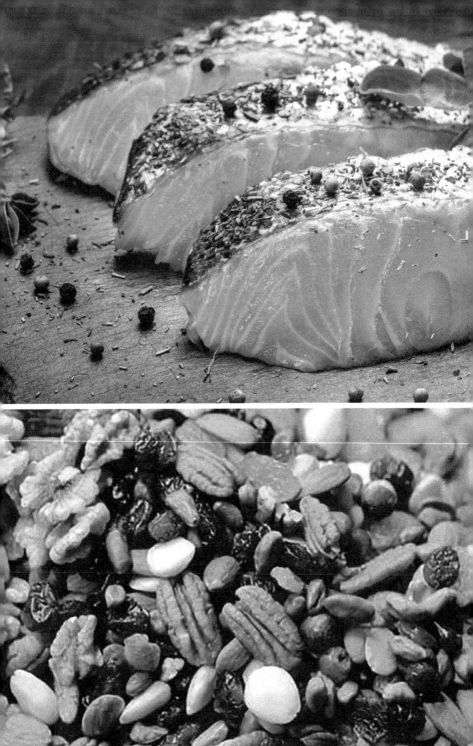

CRAMPS

MENSTRUAL - Foods to Relieve Cramps

- **Calcium** - Calcium in the diet can be an immense help in terms of cramping. However, the calcium should not be from dairy products, because that can actually trigger cramps. Other sources of calcium include **almonds, sesame seeds**, **and leafy green vegetables**. One can also use supplements but it is best to consult one's doctor first before using the supplements.

- **Dark chocolate** - Dark chocolate will not only satisfy your craving for chocolate but also help relax your muscles, and keep you happy.

- **Celery** - Celery helps with bloating and is just good for overall health as it has a lot of water and very little calories. One can enhance its taste by spreading it with peanut butter or dipping it into other foods like fruits.

- **Pineapple** - Pineapple helps in relaxing muscles, which will in turn reduce cramps. It also helps with bloating and can even boost one's mood. One can eat it plain, drink it as a juice or in a smoothie.

- **Bananas** - It is commonly said that eating a banana after exercising stops muscle cramps from settling in the next day. The same thing is true for menstrual cramps. Eat a banana before or during your cycle to avoid cramps and reduce bloating. Experts at John Hopkins University in Baltimore found that too little sleep made women more susceptible to pain (meaning those cramps will feel even worse). So make sure to get your sleep by eating bananas, which contain melatonin—a sleep-aid hormone that's secreted at night and helps regulate our body's natural rhythms[32]

- **Tea** - Caffeine should be avoided during one's period, since it can make one anxious and retain water. So, herbal tea without caffeine is best. For example, green tea can help with cramps, while peppermint tea can soothe an upset stomach.

- **Spinach and Kale** - Leafy green vegetables are one of the things one should always have in one's diet. During one's period they can help with cramps

---

32 http://www.womenshealthmag.com/food/foods-fight-pms

and be a great source of the calcium one needs. Try blending some into a smoothie with some fruit and almond milk and enjoy the taste while making sure you compliment your daily servings in the fruits, vegetables and the calcium.

- **Wheat Germ** - Wheat germ may be one of the best foods you can include in your diet if you suffer from menstrual cramps. It provides a concentrated source of **vitamin B6** (pyridoxine), with a mere cup of crude wheat germ providing a whopping 75% of the recommended daily intake for this important vitamin! **Wheat germ** is also an excellent source of other **B vitamins** as well as **zinc**. What's more, it contains very high amounts of **vitamin E and magnesium.**[33]

- **Sunflower Seeds** - Sunflower seeds are an excellent addition to your diet if you suffer from menstrual cramps. These mild nutty tasting seeds are loaded with **vitamin E** as well as the key anti-cramping minerals **zinc and magnesium.** Sunflower seeds are also an excellent source of **pyridoxine (vitamin B6)**, with one cup providing nearly a third of the recommended daily intake for this important pain relieving vitamin. The pain killing effects of **pyridoxine** may be linked to its role in the synthesis of the neurotransmitter dopamine. In addition, pyridoxine has been shown

---

[33] http://www.healwithfood.org/menstrualcramps/foods.php#ixzz3sAXRT088

to promote the absorption of **zinc** and **magnesium**. When incorporating sunflower seeds into your diet, moderation should be exercised because these seeds, like most other seeds, are high in calories and fat.

- **Parsley** - This vegetable is much more than just a decorative garnish that accompanies meals in restaurants. It is loaded with important nutrients, and it can be used to treat various health problems, including menstrual cramps. It contains **apiol,** a compound that has been shown to be highly effective at stimulating the menstrual process and relieving menstrual cramps.[34]

- **Ginger** - In traditional Chinese medicine, **ginger** has been widely used as a remedy for menstrual cramps, and a large body of anecdotal evidence from around the world validates the use of ginger as an anti-cramping remedy. Fresh ginger, which is said to be the most effective form of ginger, is available year-round in the produce section of supermarkets.[35]

- **Walnuts** - Consuming walnuts in moderation can confer great benefits to women who suffer from cramps during menstruation. Walnuts are rich in the healthy **omega-3 fatty acids** which are known to have anti-inflammatory and pain-relieving properties

---

34 http://www.healwithfood.org/menstrualcramps/foods

35 IBID

but which are often in short supply in modern diets. In addition, walnuts are loaded with **vitamin B6**, with one cup of chopped walnuts providing 31% of the recommended daily intake for this potent pain-relieving vitamin. They also contain substantial amounts of **magnesium**. Walnuts can be eaten on their own as a snack or as an ingredient in various sweet and savory dishes.

- **Sesame Seeds** - Sesame seeds are loaded with nutrients that have been shown to reduce cramps associated with menstruation, which makes them some of the best anti-cramp relievers. They are a very reliable source of **vitamin B6**, with half a cup providing more than a quarter of the recommended daily intake for this vitamin. Furthermore, they are an excellent source of plant-based **calcium** and a major source of **magnesium**. They also contain certain healthful fatty acids that may help relax muscles and thus reduce cramping further. On top of that, they provide a very reliable source of **zinc**. Sesame seeds can be added to different dishes such as salads and smoothies.

- **Oats** - Oats are loaded with the anti-cramping mineral **magnesium**. They are also one of the best sources of dietary **zinc** for women who suffer from painful periods. Before eating oats, it is advisable to soak them for several hours. Untreated oats, like other grains, contain phytic acid which can block the absorption of calcium, zinc, and magnesium in the intestines. Soaking allows enzymes to break down and neutralize phytic acid and thus improve the nutritional value of oats.[36]

· **Salmon** - This fish is full of **omega-3** and **vitamin D**, both of which help with PMS symptoms. So make sure you eat this the week before your period. It also has anti-inflammatory effects, keeping your cramps in check and reducing bloating. In fact, research from Harvard-affiliated McLean Hospital found that omega-3s are so powerful, they may even function like an antidepressant. Grilled salmon, fortified eggs, and chia seeds are all great sources to keep the menstrual blues at bay[37]

· **Water** - Drinking enough water can solve many problems. It can prevent acne, keep away cramps, and can especially help with bloating and constipation. If one is getting enough water, the body will not retain liquids and this keeps one comfortable.

---

36   http://www.healwithfood.org/menstrualcramps/food

37   http://www.womenshealthmag.com/food/foods-fight-pms

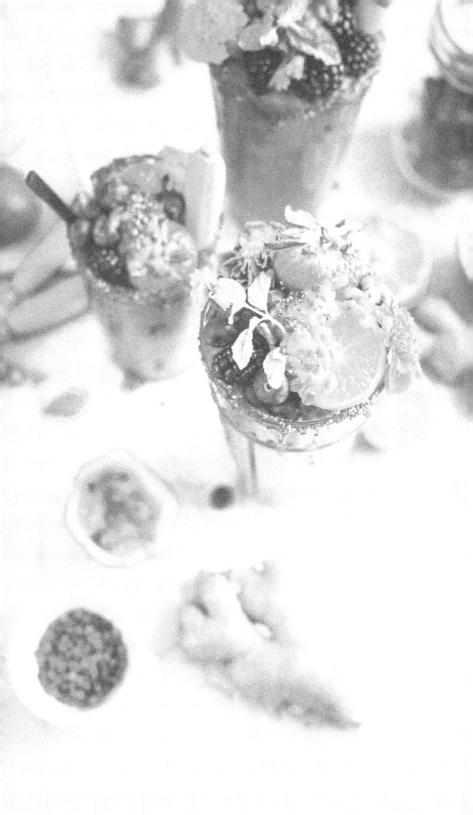

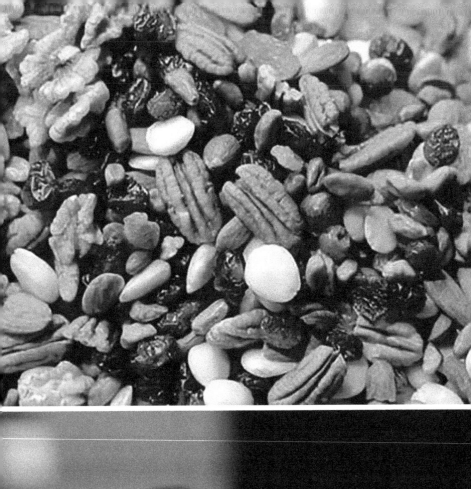
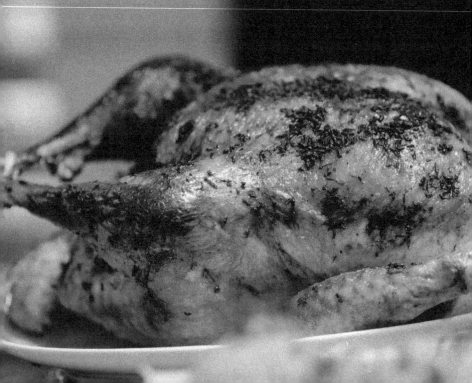

DEPRESSION

Foods That Elevate Your Mood

- **Turkey** - Most lean sources of protein are good for beating depression, but turkey has the edge due to its relatively higher levels of a chemical called **tryptophan.**[38]

- **Walnuts** - When eaten in moderation, most **nuts** are a reliable source of heart-healthy monounsaturated fats as well as protein. But walnuts get the edge when it comes to lessening the symptoms of depression because they also are one of the richest **plant-based source of omega-3 fatty acids.** "The omega-3s

---

[38] "Turkey is the best food we know of because of its tryptophan content," says Robin H-C, a life coach, behaviorist, and author of Thinking Your Way to Happy! "This chemical stimulates serotonin production, which is a natural feel-good chemical your body produces."

in walnuts support overall brain health," says Robin H-C.[39]

- **Fatty Fish** – "When it comes to omega-3 fatty acids, no food source is better than fatty fish like mackerel, bluefish, wild salmon, and tuna", says Talbott[40]. He adds that the fatty acids found in these fish not only have specific brain-boosting properties to fight depression, but also are good for overall health as well. They improve circulation and reduce inflammation and one's overall risk of heart disease.

- **Low-Fat Dairy** - Skim milk, yogurt, low-fat cheeses, and other dairy products are rich in calcium, vitamin D, and protein. These are great for your body for many reasons, including fighting depression. "Low-fat dairy is the richest dietary source of two powerhouse nutrients, calcium and vitamin D, as well as specific peptides (proteins) that induce a sense of well-being and relaxation," says Talbott[41].

39   http://www.everydayhealth.com/depression-pictures/depression-symptoms-to-watch-for.aspx

40   http://www.everydayhealth.com/drugs/omega-3-polyunsaturated-fatty-acids

41   http://www.everydayhealth.com/columns/therese-borchard-sanity-break/nutritional-deficiencies-that-may-cause-depression/

- **Whole Grains** - The high-fiber carbohydrates found in whole grains are not only healthy but can make you feel good at the same time. "Complex carbohydrates are wonderful foods to improve mood quickly," says Debbie Mandel, a stress management expert and author of Addicted to Stress. Whole grains, brown rice, oatmeal, sweet potatoes, and whole wheat pasta are all good choices. They help the body release serotonin. Some tropical grains like **sorghum and millet** are also great high fiber carbohydrates.

- **Green Tea** - Researchers know that green tea is an incredibly rich source of antioxidants, but its depression-fighting properties can be traced to an amino acid known as theanine. Theanine is an amino acid naturally found in tea leaves that provides an anti-stress relaxation benefit to tea drinkers. The presence of theanine in green tea is thought to be responsible for the observation that caffeine intake in coffee drinkers (who aren't getting theanine) is more apt to result in tension as opposed to the 'relaxed alertness' more common to tea drinkers. [42]

- **Turmeric** - This bold spice found in many Indian and Asian curry dishes is a wonderful way to boost one's mood, among other benefits. "Turmeric can indeed be considered one of the 'spices of life' because of its profound anti-inflammatory activity. Famously

---

42 http://www.everydayhealth.com/photogallery/superfoods.aspx

used in spicy Indian and Thai dishes, turmeric contains the active compounds turmerones and curcuminoids, which have been associated with a wide range of health benefits," says Talbott.

- **Dark chocolate** helps to release serotonin and relaxes the blood vessels of the cardiovascular system.. Just remember that dark chocolate is incredibly calorie-dense, with about 150 calories per ounce, so eat just one small piece at a time.[43]

- **Dark Leafy Greens** - Dark Leafy Greens can easily be considered the healthiest food of all, the most nutrient-dense item available to us to eat. Examples are **Spinach. Kale and Swiss chard**. Greens are the first of the G-BOMBS (Greens, Beans, Onions, Mushrooms, Berries, Seeds) that Dr. Fuhrman describes in his book, The End of Dieting the foods with the most powerful immune-boosting and anticancer effect.

"These foods help to prevent the cancerous transformation of normal cells and keep the body armed and ready to attack any precancerous or cancerous cells that may arise," Dr. Fuhrman writes. They fight against all kinds of inflammation, and according to a new study published in JAMA Psychiatry, severe depression has been linked

---

43 IBID

with brain inflammation. Leafy greens are especially important because they contain lots of vitamin A.

- **Avocados** are power foods because they contain healthy fat that our brains need to run smoothly. Three-fourths of the calories of an avocado are from fat, mostly monounsaturated fat, in the form of oleic acid. An average avocado also contains 4 grams of protein, higher than other fruits, and is filled with vitamin K, different kinds of vitamin B (B-9, B-6, and B-5), vitamin C, and vitamin E-12. Finally, they are low in sugar and high in dietary fiber, containing about 11 grams each.

- **Berries - Blueberries, raspberries, strawberries**, and **blackberries** are some of the highest antioxidant foods available to us. In a study published in the Journal of Nutritional and Environmental Medicine[44], patients were treated for two years with antioxidants or placebos. After two years those who were treated with antioxidants had a significantly lower depression score. They are like DNA repairmen. They go around fixing your cells and preventing them from getting cancer and other illnesses.

---

44 http://www.researchgate.net/publication/232044373_Impact_
of_Antioxidant_Therapy_on_Symptoms_of_Anxiety_and_
Depression._A_Randomized_Controlled_Trial_in_Patients_with_
Peripheral_Arterial_Disease

- **Mushrooms** - Here are two good reasons why mushrooms are good for your mental health. First, their chemical properties oppose insulin, which helps lower blood sugar levels, evening out your mood. They also are like a probiotic in that they promote healthy gut bacteria. And since the nerve cells in our gut manufacture 80 percent to 90 percent of our body's serotonin — the critical neurotransmitter that keeps us sane — we can't afford to not pay attention to our intestinal health.

- **Tomatoes** - Tomatoes contain lots of folic acid and alpha-lipoic acid, both of which are good for fighting depression. According to research published in the Journal of Psychiatry and Neuroscience.[45] Many studies show an elevated incidence of folate deficiency in patients with depression. In most of the studies, about one-third of depression patients were deficient in folate.

Folic acid can prevent an excess of homocysteine — which restricts the production of important neurotransmitters like serotonin, dopamine, and norepinephrine — from forming in the body. This helps the body convert glucose into energy, and therefore stabilizes mood.

- **Beans** - Beans make the G-BOMB list because they can act as anti-diabetes and weight-loss foods. They

---

45 http://www.ncbi.nlm.nih.gov/pmc/articles/PMC1810582/

are good for our moods because our bodies digest them slowly, which stabilizes blood sugar levels. Any food that assists in evening out blood sugar levels is good for us.

- **Seeds** - Seeds are the last food on Fuhrman's G-BOMBS list. **Flaxseeds, hemp seeds,** and **chia seeds** are especially good for one's mood because they are rich in omega-3 fatty acids. Fuhrman writes, "Not only do seeds add their own spectrum of unique disease-fighting substances to the dietary landscape, but the fat in seeds increases the absorption of protective nutrients in vegetables eaten at the same meal."

- **Apples** - Like berries, **apples** are high in antioxidants, which can help to prevent and repair oxidation damage and inflammation on the cellular level. They are also full of soluble fiber, which balances blood sugar swings.

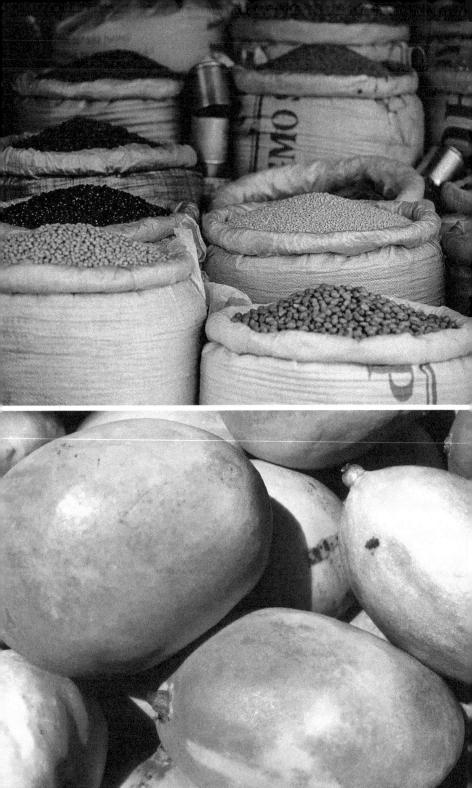

DIABETES[46]

Foods to Balance Blood Sugar

- **Vitamin C** - A European study found that people with the most vitamin C in their bodies had the lowest incidence of diabetes, although the link isn't clear. **Fruits and veggies like oranges, strawberries, and broccoli** are the best sources of Vitamin C.

- **Mangoes** - Not only the fruit but the leaves of mangoes are healthy too. For people suffering from diabetes, just boil 5-6 mango leaves in a vessel, soak it through the night and drink the filtered decoction in the morning. This helps in regulating your insulin levels.[47]

---

46 http://www.besthealthmag.ca/best-you/diabetes/
the-top-20-foods-for-beating-diabetes

47 https://healthimpactnews.
com/2013/17-reasons-why-you-need-a-mango-every-day/

- **Spices** - Researchers from the University of Georgia tested 24 common herbs and spices and discovered that their antioxidants could prevent inflammation associated with diabetes. **Cloves** and **cinnamon** both got high rankings.[48]

- **Brown Rice** - A compound that helps the rice grow reduces nerve and blood vessel damage from diabetes, according to the Medical College of Georgia experts. Soak the dry rice in water overnight, which awakens the compound.

- **Apples** - Because they offer so many health advantages, put these at the core of your diet. Apples are naturally low in calories, yet their high fibre content (4 grams) fills you up, battles bad cholesterol, and blunts blood-sugar swings. Red Delicious and Granny Smith are also among the top 10 fruits with the most disease-fighting antioxidants. Eaten whole and unpeeled they provide the greatest benefit.[49]

- **Avocado** - Avocado slows digestion and helps keep blood sugar from spiking after a meal. A diet high in good fats may even help reverse insulin resistance, which translates to steadier blood sugar

---

48 Ibid

49 http://www.besthealthmag.ca/eat-well/
nutrition/15-health-benefits-of-eating-apples

in the long-term. Try putting mashed avocado on sandwiches instead of mayonnaise or on bread instead of butter. [50]

- **Barley** - Choosing this grain instead of white rice can reduce the rise in blood sugar after a meal by almost 70 per cent—and keep your blood sugar lower and steadier for hours. That's because the soluble fibre and other compounds in barley dramatically slow the digestion and absorption of the carbohydrate. Other whole grains like **sorghum** and **millet** have similar effects.

- **Beans** - Add beans to your diet at least twice a week. The soluble fibre in all types of beans prevents high blood sugar. And because they're rich in protein, beans can stand in for meat in main dishes. Just watch the sodium content, especially from baked beans. Soaked beans are tender in just 10 to 15 minutes.

- **Berries** - Berries are full of fibre and antioxidants. The red and blue varieties also contain natural plant compounds called anthocyanins. Scientists believe these may help lower blood sugar by boosting insulin production.

- **Broccoli** - Broccoli is filling, fibrous, and full of antioxidants and vitamin C. It's also rich in **chromium**, which plays a key role in long-term blood

50 IBID

sugar control. For those who do not particularly fancy it, you can "hide" it in smoothies, soups, pasta dishes, and casseroles, or sauté it with garlic, soy sauce, and mustard, or dark sesame oil.

· **Carrots** - While the type of sugar they contain is transformed into blood sugar quickly, the amount of sugar in carrots is extremely low. That's good because carrots are one of nature's richest sources of beta-carotene, which is linked to a lower risk of diabetes and better blood-sugar control.

· **Chicken or turkey** - For best results, breast meat, whether ground or whole, is always lower in fat than dark meat such as thighs and drumsticks. The skin should be avoided because of its high saturated fat content. Roasting your meat is best.

· **Eggs** - Egg protein is the gold standard nutritionists use to rank all other proteins because eggs are another excellent, inexpensive source of high-quality protein—so high, in fact, that they raise your cholesterol, and will keep you feeling full and satisfied for hours afterward.

· **Fish** - The single deadliest complication of diabetes is heart disease, and eating fish just once a week can reduce your risk by 40 per cent, according to a Harvard School of Public Health study. The fatty acids in fish reduce inflammation in the body - a major contributor to coronary disease, as well as insulin resistance and diabetes.

- **Flax Seeds** - Flax Seeds are a source of magnesium, a mineral that's key to blood-sugar control because it helps cells use insulin. Sprinkle on cereal, yoghurt, or ice cream or blend into meatballs, burgers, pancakes, breads and smoothies.

- **Milk and yogurt** - Both are rich in protein and calcium, which studies show may help people lose weight. And diets that include plenty of dairy may fight insulin resistance, a core problem behind diabetes. Go low-fat or fat-free.

- **Nuts** - Because of their high fibre and protein content, nuts are "slow burning" foods that are friendly to blood sugar. And even though they contain a lot of fat, it's that healthful monounsaturated kind. Roasting really brings out the flavour of nuts and makes them a great addition to fall soups and entrées.

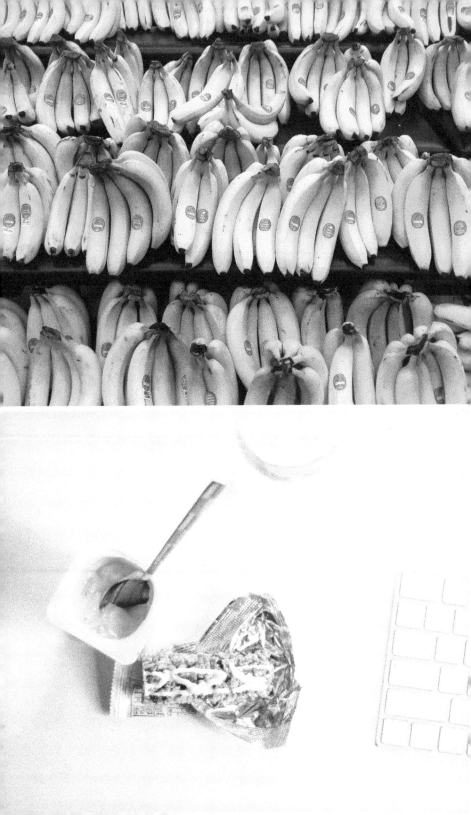

DIARRHEA

Foods to Relieve Diarrhea

Unlike the other foods in this book which are for prevention, the ones here for diarrhea are more for prompt home remedies or for lessening the symptoms at the time. When your stomach is acting up, it could be because you ate the wrong things, maybe you are under stress, or maybe you have absolutely no idea why your stomach is feeling so lousy. It is hard to know what to eat without making things worse.

The basic BRAT diet (bananas, rice, applesauce, and toast) is a good start. Here is a quick guide as to why the BRAT diet helps, as well as some other choices that are safe and soothing.[51]

---

51 By Barbara Bolen, PhD - Reviewed by a board of certified physicians in https://www.verywell.com/ibs-4014702. Updated August 31, 2016

- **Bananas** - Bland and easily digested, bananas are an excellent choice to settle an upset digestive system. The elevated level of potassium in bananas helps to replace electrolytes that may be lost by severe bouts of diarrhea. Bananas are also rich in pectin, a soluble fiber that helps to absorb liquid in the intestines and thus move the stool along smoothly.

Bananas also contain a good amount of inulin, another soluble fiber. Inulin is a prebiotic, a substance that promotes the growth of beneficial bacteria (probiotics) in the intestinal system.

- **Applesauce** - Like bananas, apples are a reliable source of pectin. However, the high fiber in raw apples makes them too rough for a dicey intestinal system.

Cooking the apples makes them easier on your system to digest. This allows you to benefit from the pectin, sugar, and other nutrients that lie within.

- **Mashed Potatoes** - Due to their low-fiber content, white potatoes are easily digested way up high in the GI tract. The potatoes should be eaten plain; butter has a high fat content, which could be irritating to one's system and contribute to intestinal cramping.

- **White Rice** - Similar to mashed potatoes, plain white rice is also easy on your digestive system. Rice also has a reputation for being "binding," which means that it can help to firm up your loose stool.

- **Steamed Chicken** - Due to its bland nature, steamed white meat chicken is an easily digested source of protein. This provides a safe way to get some nutrients into your body. Butter and oils are very hard on a delicate system, so avoid deep-fried or sautéed preparations.

- **Yogurt** - It is generally recommended that dairy products be avoided during acute diarrhea episodes. Yogurt is a major exception to this rule. Look for yogurt that contains live or active cultures, or more specifically *Lactobacillus acidophilus* and *Bifidobacterium bifidum*. These active cultures are probiotics and they appear to help establish a healthier balance of bacteria in the digestive tract. Read the label carefully and choose a brand that does not have a high sugar level or does not contain artificial sweeteners. Both of those can contribute to excessive intestinal gas and loose stools.

- **Blueberries** - Reportedly, dried blueberries have a long history of use in Sweden as a treatment for diarrhea. Dr. Varro Tyler in his book, *"Herbs of Choice,"* recommends either chewing dried blueberries or making a tea by boiling crushed dried blueberries for about 10 minutes. The helpfulness of blueberries for diarrhea appears to be due to the fact that they contain tannins, which act as an astringent, contracting tissue and reducing inflammation and secretion of liquids and mucus. Blueberries also contain substances called anthocyanosides, which have antibacterial properties, as well as being a reliable source of antioxidants. Lastly, blueberries are another source of the soluble fiber pectin.

- **Peppermint Tea** - Peppermint has a soothing effect on the gastrointestinal system. It is thought to calm and relax the muscles along the intestinal tract, thus reducing spasms. Peppermint also seems to be effective in reducing intestinal gas.

Tropical

Guava leaves are herbal medicine for dysentery & diarrhea. To treat diarrhea, you will have to boil 30 grams of guava leaves with a handful of rice flour in one glass water and drink this solution twice a day

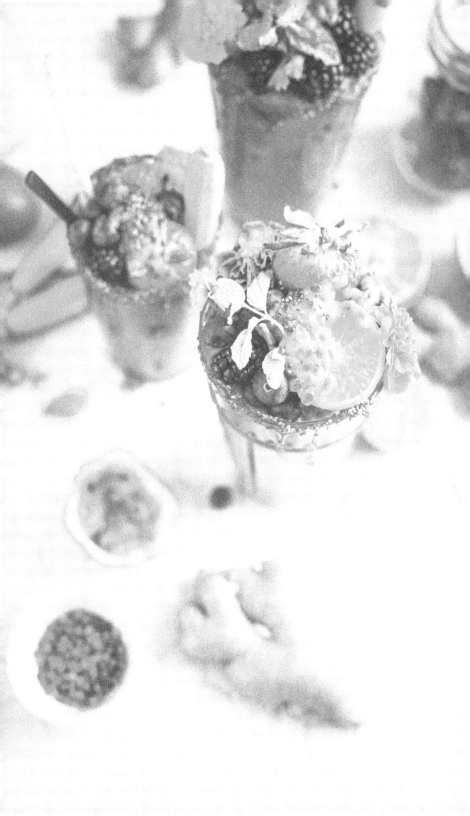

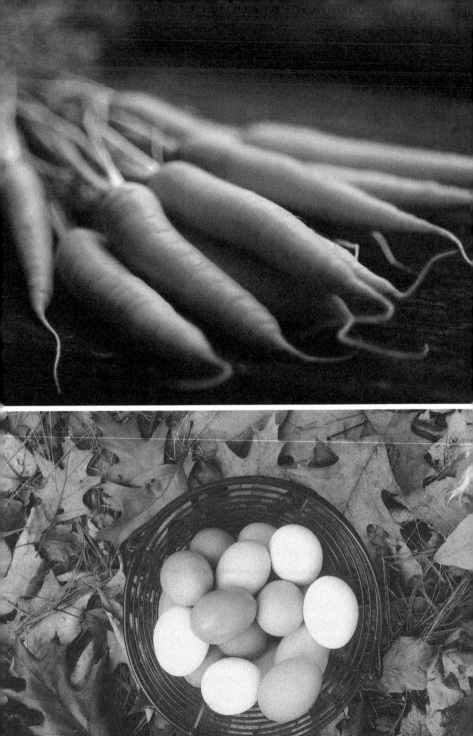

EYESIGHT

Foods to Improve Eyesight[52]

- **Fish** - Cold-water fish such as salmon, tuna, sardines and mackerel are rich in omega-3 fatty acids, which may help protect against dry eyes, macular degeneration and even cataracts. If you don't eat seafood, you can get a good supply of omega-3s by using **fish oil supplements** or taking vegetarian supplements that contain **black currant seed oil or flaxseed oil.**

- **Leafy Greens** - **Spinach, kale** and **collard greens**, to name a few, are full of lutein and zeaxanthin, plant pigments that can help stem the development of macular degeneration and cataracts. **Broccoli, peas** and **avocados** are also reliable sources of this

---

52 http://www.health.harvard.edu/staying-healthy/
top-foods-to-help-protect-your-vision

powerful antioxidant duo. Rich in cancer-fighting antioxidants and vitamins, **kale** is also a good source of beta-carotene and is the top combo of both lutein and zeaxanthin; one cup of greens contains 23.8 mg of lutein and zeaxanthin. Use kale in a salad or a side dish; blend it into fruit smoothies; or bake the leaves into kale chips[53]

- **Eggs** - The vitamins and nutrients in eggs, including lutein and vitamin A (which may protect against night blindness and dry eyes), promote eye health and function.

- **Whole Grains** - A diet containing foods with a low glycemic index (GI) can help reduce your risk for age-related macular degeneration.

Swap refined carbohydrates for quinoa, brown rice, whole oats and whole-wheat breads and pasta. The vitamin E, zinc and niacin found in whole grains also help promote overall eye health. **Corn** also contains some lutein and zeaxanthin. Research in the Journal of Agricultural Food and Chemistry discovered that cooking this veggie longer increased the amount of lutein and the antioxidant levels per serving. Add it to chilis, soups, and casseroles.[54]

---

53 http://www.rd.com/health/wellness/
   improve-your-eyesight-foods-to-eat/

54 http://www.rd.com/health/wellness/
   improve-your-eyesight-foods-to-eat/

- **Citrus Fruits and Berries - Oranges, grapefruits, lemons and berries** are high in vitamin C, which may reduce the risk of cataracts and macular degeneration.

- **Nuts - Pistachios, walnuts, almonds** are rich in omega-3 fatty acids and vitamin E that boost eye health.

- **Colorful Fruits and Vegetables** - Foods such as **carrots, tomatoes, bell peppers, strawberries, pumpkin, corn** and **cantaloupe** are excellent sources of vitamins A and C and carotenoids, the compounds that give these fruits and vegetables their yellow, orange and red pigments. These are thought to help decrease the risk of many eye diseases.

- **Legumes - Kidney beans, black-eyed peas and lentils** are reliable sources of bioflavonoids and zinc and can help protect the retina and lower the risk for developing macular degeneration and cataracts.

- **Fish Oil, Flaxseed Oil and Black Currant Seed Oil**

These super supplements contain omega-3 fatty acids and have many eye health benefits, including helping to prevent or control dry eye syndrome as well as reduce the risk of macular degeneration and cataracts.

- **Sunflower Seeds** - Help keep your eyes healthy and disease-free by snacking on sunflower seeds, which are excellent sources of vitamin E and zinc.

- **Beef** - In moderation, lean beef in your diet can boost your eye health. Beef contains zinc, which helps your body absorb vitamin A and may play a role in reducing risk of advanced age-related macular degeneration.

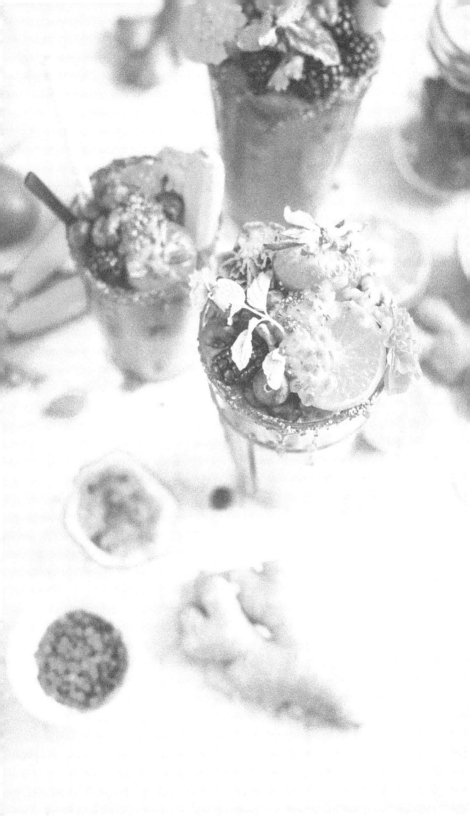

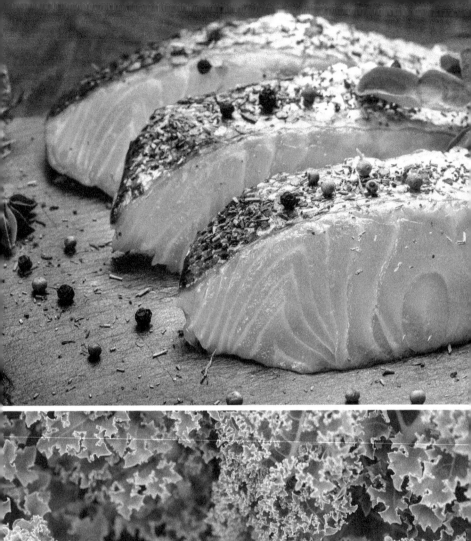
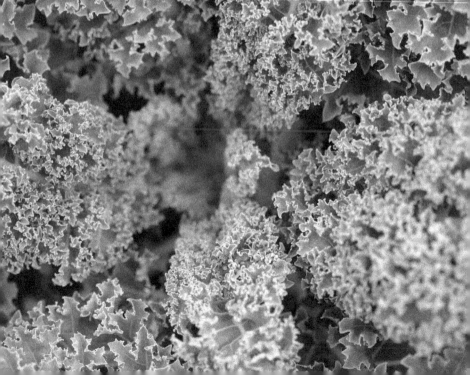

FERTILITY

Foods to Enhance Fertility[55]

- **Walnuts - because of Omega 6 & 3**

- **Oysters**, because of best source of zinc, selenium, Vitamin B12, iron

- **Pomegranates** - high concentration of Vitamin C

- **Brazil nuts**

- **Garlic** is a great conception booster for men. It contains allicin, which improves blood flow to his sexual organs and protects sperm from damage, and selenium, an antioxidant that improves sperm quality.

- **Vegetables and Fruits** - Studies have also shown organic vegetables and fruits to have more nutritional value. A **banana** should be your go-to mid-morning

55 http://www.health.harvard.edu/diseases-and-conditions/
    follow-fertility-diet

snack if you're trying for a baby. Each one is packed with vitamin B6, which regulates the hormones and is needed for good egg and sperm development[56].

- **Cold water fish** - Fish supplies important essential fatty acids (omega 3) to our diet. These fatty acids aid in the production of hormones, reduce inflammation, and help regulate the menstrual cycle. Fish is also a great source of protein and vitamin A. One should avoid large deep water fish such as tuna, swordfish, and Chilean sea bass due to their potential concentrations of mercury, and focus on cold water fish such as wild salmon, cod, and halibut.

- **Grains in their whole, natural form** - Whole grains are filled with fiber, important vitamins, and immune supporting properties. Fiber is important for helping the body to get rid of excess hormones and helps to keep the blood sugar balanced. Avoid processed and refined white foods and grains such as white bread, semolina pastas, and white rice. Instead choose whole wheat or sprouted bread, rice or whole wheat pasta, quinoa, and brown rice.

- **Chicken** - Protein is important for your egg production – and gram for gram chicken is a great source. But hold off on that Atkins diet while

---

56 http://www.motherandbaby.co.uk/trying-for-a-baby/
pregnancy-planning/help-to-get-pregnant

trying to conceive, as high-protein diets aren't advised pre-pregnancy.

- **Eat high fiber foods with each meal** - Fiber helps to regulate blood sugar levels which helps to reduce fertility issues such as PCOS, immunological issues, and promotes healthy hormonal balance. Some examples of high fiber foods are **fruits, vegetables, dark leafy greens, and beans.**

- **Eggs**- Eggs contain vitamin D, thought to help increase fertility levels in women. The protein in eggs also make them an ideal breakfast for someone trying to get pregnant.

- **Vitamin C**: Vitamin C improves hormone levels and increases fertility in women with luteal phase defect, according to a study published in *Fertility and Sterility*. As for men, vitamin C has been shown to improve sperm quality and protect sperm from DNA damage; helping to reduce the chance of miscarriage and chromosomal problems. Vitamin C also appears to keep sperm from clumping together, making them more motile. Food sources: Abundant in **plants and fruits** including **red peppers, broccoli, cranberries, cabbage, potatoes, tomatoes, and citrus fruits.**

A Harvard Medical School research done recently showed an 80% decrease in infertility with lifestyle changes made by switching to a fertility diet. Women who followed a combination of five or more lifestyle factors, including changing specific aspects of their diets, experienced more than 80 percent less relative risk of infertility due to ovulatory disorders compared to women who engaged in none of the factors, according to a paper published in *Obstetrics & Gynecology.*[57]

The women with the highest fertility diet scores ate **less trans fats and sugar** from carbohydrates, consumed **more protein from vegetables than from animals**, ate **more fiber and iron, took more multivitamins,** had a lower body mass index (BMI), **exercised for longer periods of time each day**, and, surprisingly, consumed more high-fat dairy products and less low-fat dairy products. The relationship between a higher "fertility diet" score and lesser risk for infertility was similar for different subgroups of women regardless of age and whether they had been pregnant in the past.[58]

Tropical

Guavas are high in vitamin A, so it makes an excellent food to protect and improve vision health. If you eat a diet rich in guava, you may be able to keep the development of macular degeneration and cataracts at bay.

---

57 http://natural-fertility-info.com/

58 IBID

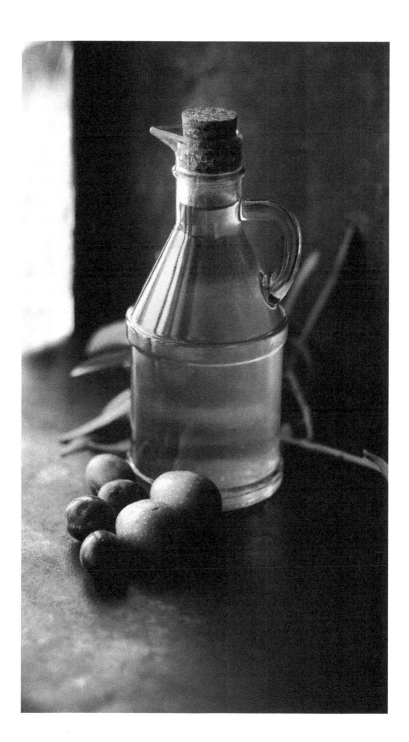

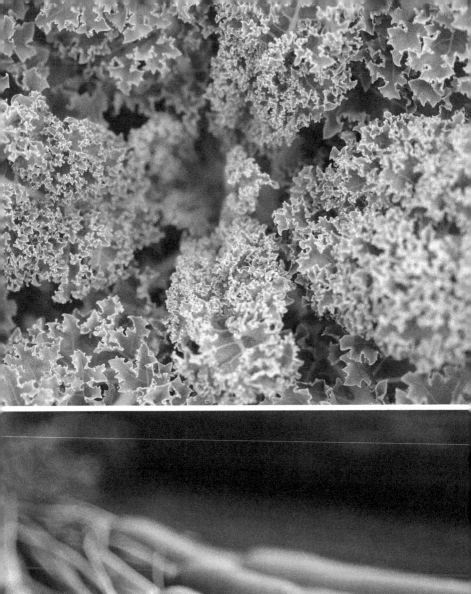
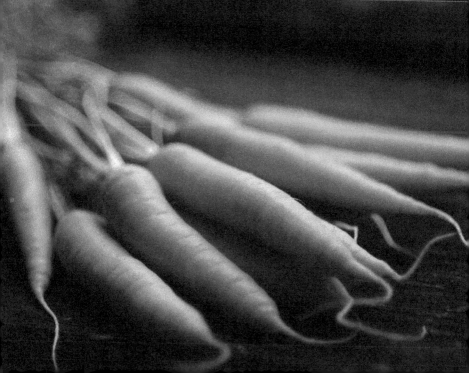

FIBROIDS[59]

Foods to Shrink Fibroids

Fibroids are extremely common. In fact, about 75 percent of women experience them at some point in their lives and they are responsible for more than 200,000 hysterectomies each year.

Fibroids are non-cancerous tumors found within the uterine walls, often resulting in a change in the size or shape of the uterus as well as several unpleasant symptoms. However, they can also be symptomless. So, whether you know you have fibroids or not, it's a great idea for any woman to do things to naturally prevent these common growths in the uterus.

Studies have shown that avoiding high blood pressure lowers the risk of developing fibroids. According to research from the Harvard Medical School and Harvard

---

59 https://draxe.com/fibroids/

School of Public Health, there is a strong and independent association between blood pressure and risk for fibroids in premenopausal women.[60]

Some risk factors for fibroids are out of one's control, but there are many one can manage. These include things like eating higher-quality beef, eating more leafy green vegetables and drinking less alcohol.

Foods to Eat

The following foods should be included in your diet to keep your fibroids at bay:

- **Organic Foods.** Eating organic foods can help to prevent and shrink fibroids. Pesticides impact estrogen and other hormone levels. Since hormonal balance is key to natural fibroid treatment, you want to reduce your pesticide intake as much as possible.

- **Green Leafy Vegetables.** Green leafy vegetables discourage the growth of fibroids in a woman's body. These vegetables are vitamin K-rich foods. This vitamin aids in clotting and helps control of menstrual bleeding.

- **Cruciferous Vegetables.** Cruciferous vegetables support detoxification of your liver and balance estrogen levels. Research has shown that high

---

60 http://www.medscape.org/viewarticle/502862_6

consumption of **broccoli, cabbage, Chinese cabbage, tomato** and **apple** seems to be a protective factor for uterine fibroids. A greater intake of cruciferous vegetables (and fresh fruits) is believed to be capable of reducing the incidence of uterine fibroids in women.[61]

- **Beta-carotene Rich Foods**. Upon digestion, the human body turns beta carotene into vitamin A, which promotes the growth of healthy tissues as well as the repair of tissues, which can both be very helpful for healing fibroids. Some foods high in beta-carotene include **carrots, sweet potatoes, kale and spinach.**

- **High-Iron Foods** - Fibroids sometimes cause some women to lose more blood during their monthly menstruation. This can lead to anemia. To replace the excessive loss of iron, include high-iron foods like **grass-fed beef** and **legumes** in your diet to help replace that lost iron and prevent anemia.

- **Flaxseeds** - Flaxseeds help balance estrogen levels in the body, which can help to shrink fibroids. One should aim for at least two tablespoons per day if one has fibroids. One can sprinkle flaxseeds on oatmeal, in smoothies or simply eat the seeds by themselves.

- **Whole Grains** - Instead of refined grains, opt for healthier whole grains, including sorghum and millet

---

61   http://www.ncbi.nlm.nih.gov/pubmed/26458740

- **Fish Oil (1,000 milligrams daily) or Flaxseed Oil (1 tablespoon daily).** The essential fatty acids found in fish oil and flaxseed oil can help reduce inflammation in your body, which may play a part in fibroid growth.

- **B-complex (50 milligrams daily)** - If B vitamins are lacking in the diet, the liver is missing some of the raw materials it needs to carry out its metabolic processes and regulate estrogen levels.

- **Herbal Teas** - Herbal teas help soothe the symptoms of fibroids by decreasing inflammation and rebalancing certain hormones. Teas made with chaste berry, milk thistle, yellow dock, dandelion root, nettle and red raspberry all have systemic benefits for the uterus and reproductive system.

- **Avoid Exposure to Environmental Toxins** - Stay clear of the following to improve your hormonal health as well as your general health: pesticides, herbicides, synthetic fertilizers, bleach, food preservatives, harmful cleaners (even certain eco-cleaners) and food dyes. You'll also want to opt for natural, unbleached feminine care products as well as organic body care products and makeup.

- **Exercise** - Getting regular exercise can help to prevent fibroids before they start! According to one study, the more a woman exercises, the less likely she is to get uterine fibroids.[62]

Avoid the following Foods:

High-Fat, Processed Meats. High-fat, **processed meats** are some of the worst food choices for women when it comes to fibroids. Foods high in unhealthy fats like non-organic meats or processed meats can increase inflammation levels and often contain chemical additives. (e.g. **hamburgers and processed breakfast sausages**).

Conventional Dairy. Non-organic dairy is very high in steroids and other chemicals that can alter hormones and encourage the development and growth of fibroids.

Refined Sugar. Consuming refined sugar can increase pain and reduce immune function in the body. It may also lead to weight gain and hormonal imbalance, two factors that encourage the development of fibroids. Studies have even shown that a high dietary glycemic index is associated with higher risk of uterine fibroids in some women.[63]

Refined Carbohydrates. Managing hormones not only involves the elimination of sugars from the diet, but also refined carbohydrates. Refined carbs cause insulin levels to spike and hormones to become out of control. Consuming

---

62 http://www.uofmhealth.org/health-library/hw183462#hw183603

63 http://www.ncbi.nlm.nih.gov/pubmed/20200259

processed grains like those in instant hot cereals and commercial breads causes a sharp rise in insulin. These refined carbohydrates have been stripped of everything but starch, so they offer negative health consequences and no good nutritional value.

Alcohol. Overdoing it in the alcohol department increases inflammation throughout the body, reduces immune function and encourages hormonal imbalances. By reducing or eliminating alcohol, you can help to get your hormones back on track and hopefully shrink those fibroids fast.

Caffeine. Too much caffeine is taxing on your body, especially your liver. When you give your liver more work to do than it ideally should have, it isn't going to do as good of a job at keeping your hormones in check. Drinking more than two cups of coffee daily may boost estrogen levels in women and could worsen conditions with a hormonal basis like fibroids.

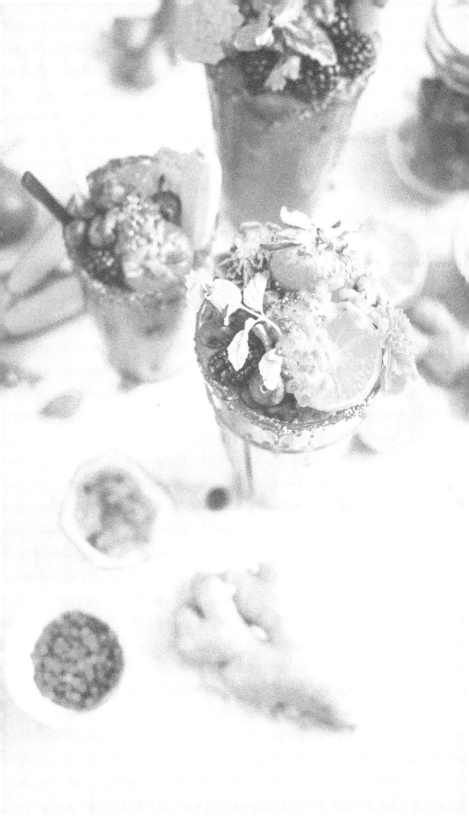

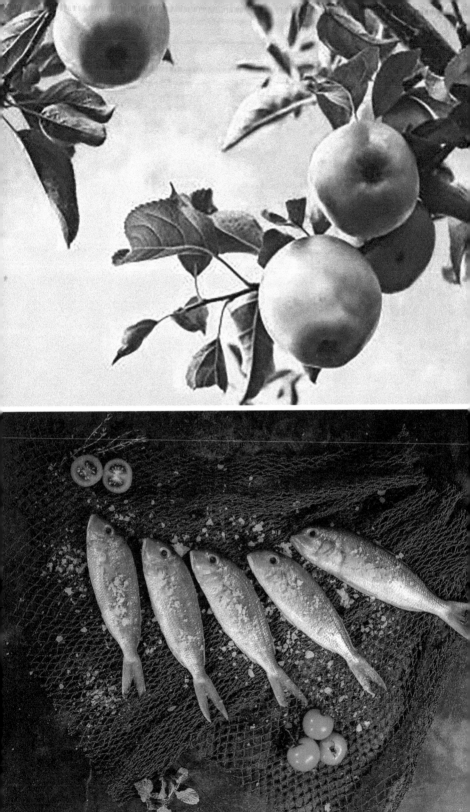

HERPES OUTBREAKS
Foods to Abate Breakouts[64]

- Eat foods rich in **lysine - Fish, chicken, beef, lamb, milk, cheese, beans, brewer's yeast, mung bean sprouts,** and most **fruits and vegetables** have more lysine than arginine, except for peas. (Arginine competes with lysine for absorption; herpes virus loves arginine and is thwarted by lysine.

- **Fruits** - Eating fruit is a great way to get adequate lysine into your body. Plenty of autumn fruits contain high amounts of lysine. Try including **apples, figs** and **pears** in your diet. Summer treats like **mangoes** and **apricots** are also beneficial.

- **Vegetables** - Research has shown that **cauliflower, Brussel sprouts** and **broccoli** are three of the best

---

64 http://www.livestrong.com/
    article/282430-foods-to-avoid-and-vitamins-for-herpes/

foods to eat to prevent a herpes outbreak. Most vegetables are high in lysine and low in arginine. **Beans, beets** and **potatoes** are other vegetables rich in lysine that you can include in your diet.

- **Dairy** - Consuming dairy products when you are suffering from herpes will help cure your sores fast. **Yoghurt** has one of the highest amounts of lysine of all foods. Make sure you eat yogurt that doesn't contain gelatin or corn syrup. Gelatin has arginine, which may cause outbreaks.

- **Meats** - Eating various types of meats can help cure your herpes. **Beef, lamb, fish** and **chicken** are all rich in lysine.

- **Adding lemon to water** is a fast way to improve the alkaline balance in your diet. Acidic foods are known to cause herpes outbreaks. Avoid taking caffeinated drinks while you have a herpes outbreak, as caffeine increases your acid level.

- **Stress-relieving foods** - Stress is a common trigger for herpes outbreaks. Luckily, some foods can decrease stress levels, especially those rich in **B vitamins** like brown rice, bananas, barley, sorghum, millet, mushrooms, turkey, salmon and tuna. Also, eat foods rich in **antioxidants** regularly, including **berries, lemon, carrots, ginger, green tea, whole grains, barley grass, goji berries, and spirulina.**

Foods to Avoid

In the 2007 edition of "Integrative Medicine," University of Wisconsin professor David Rakel, M.D. recommends steering clear of foods rich in the amino acid arginine, such as **chocolate, peanuts, cashews, almonds, sunflower seeds and gelatin**. According to Dr. Rakel, the herpes simplex virus requires arginine to reproduce. Diets high in arginine can trigger the virus to begin reproducing. Although arginine is found in many foods, including meat, poultry, fish, dairy products and legumes, arginine in these foods is counteracted by another amino acid, lysine, that opposes the effects of arginine on the herpes simplex virus[65]

---

65 http://www.livestrong.com/
article/282430-foods-to-avoid-and-vitamins-for-herpes

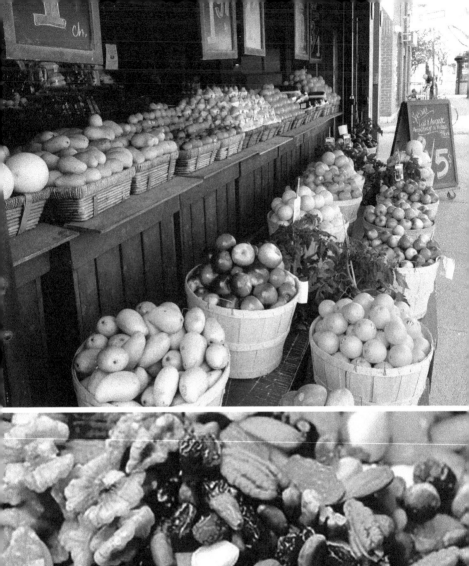
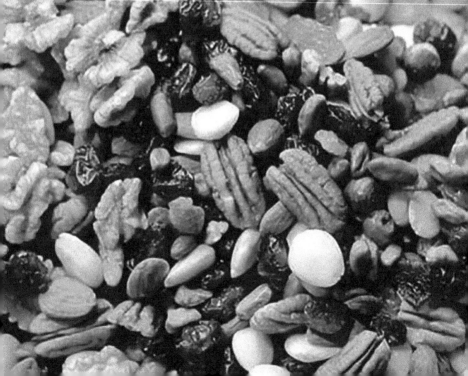

HIV & AIDS

Foods to Support Immunity

If you have HIV, and you are getting treatment and not having complications, then eat the same healthy diet that everyone should be eating.[66]

The general principles of healthy eating are simple:

- Eat lots of **fruits and vegetables** (7 to 8 servings a day).[67]

- Favor **whole grains**, which provide fiber and healthy nutrients.

- Choose lean proteins, such as **fish, chicken, beans, legumes, and low-fat dairy.**

- Select healthier fats, in moderate servings, like **olive oil, nuts** and **avocados**

---

66 http://www.webmd.com/hiv-aids/default.htm

67 Canada's Food Guide

- **Limit sugar**, **sweets**, and **saturated fats.**

- **Skip trans fats** totally.

- **Avoid fad diets** - Extreme diets that cut out whole food groups or advise taking huge doses of vitamins or supplements may be dangerous.

- Eat for your general health, not just HIV. Don't focus only on a special immunity-boosting diet if it could hurt your all-around health. People with HIV may be at higher risk for heart disease, cancer, osteoporosis, and other conditions, but a good overall diet can help prevent them.

- Keep it simple. The more complex a diet becomes, the more difficult it is to follow. Some people try to measure their intake of protein and fat down to the ounce. But unless there's a specific medical reason, most people don't need to worry about that level of detail, says Kimberly Dong, RD, a dietitian at Tufts University School of Medicine.

- Get help if you have problems. A normal healthy diet is good for most people with HIV. But if you are having problems - like a loss of appetite, nausea, or unwanted weight loss, see your doctor. Don't try to deal with it on your own. Your doctor can help treat both the underlying problem and the symptoms.

It is recommended that the diet for HIV-positive persons and AIDS patients be rich in **whole, natural foods, such** as fruits, vegetables, grains, beans, seeds and nuts; low in fats and refined sugars and adequate amounts of protein. Also, supplementing with zinc and selenium, antioxidants, such as Vitamin C and E, is useful in addressing the wasting syndrome and healing the gastrointestinal tract.[68]

One way to remember the eating guidelines is the U.S. government's "MyPlate" recommendation: Make half your plate vegetables and fruits, and split the other half between grains and protein.[69]

---

68   Foods that fight disease" by Leslie Beck RD, Penguin Canada

69   http://www.webmd.com/food-recipes/guide/
     myplate-food-groups-and-portions

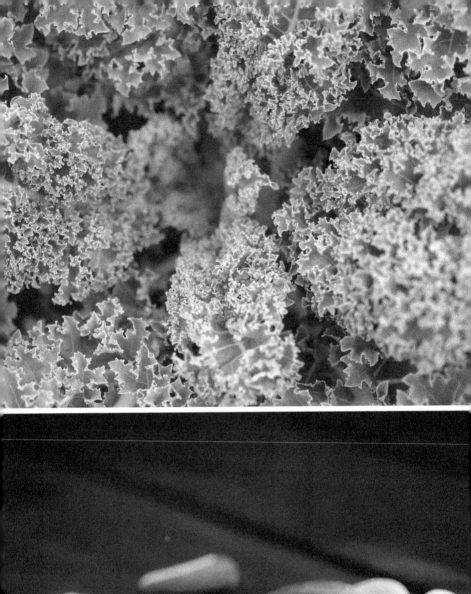
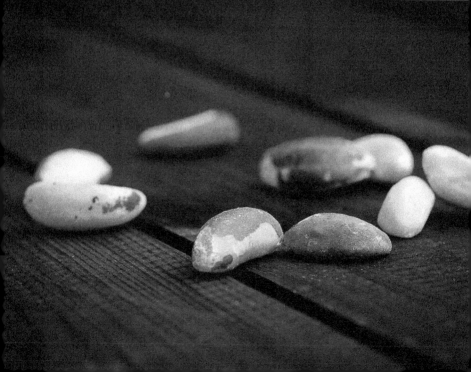

HOT FLASHES.

Foods to Cool Hot Flashes

To create better health and hormonal balance and reduce hot flashes tap into the endless variety of **plant based foods** A balanced diet of **quality protein, healthy fats**, and **phytonutrient-rich fruits** and **vegetables, together with regular exercise, adequate sleep and stress reduction**, are all that is needed to regulate healthy hormonal and neurotransmitter balance in most women. You can also take a top-quality **multivitamin-mineral complex and omega-3 supplement**, not only to ensure that your nutritional bases are covered for today and tomorrow, but that the inevitable swings of hormonal change are less dramatic and unpleasant

- **Soy** - Research indicates that **soy**, a significant element in the traditional Japanese diet, may be useful in preventing hot flashes in women. Edible beans, especially **soybeans**, contain the compounds

genistein and daidzein, which are estrogenic and help control hot flashes. That may explain why only 7 percent of menopausal Japanese women suffer from hot flashes, as compared to 55 percent of women living in the United States, according to Dr. Lindsey Berkson's estimates in "Hormone Deception." "Besides providing more vegetable protein and less animal protein than a Western diet, it's also low in fat and high in soy products such as tofu. These foods are rich in plant compounds known as phytoestrogens, which seem to mimic some of the biological activities of female hormones."[70]

- **Calcium-rich foods** - In addition to **soy and tofu products**, women can help combat hot flashes by eating more **calcium-rich foods, magnesium-rich foods** and **foods rich in vitamin E - like cold-pressed oils, green leafy vegetables, nuts and almonds**, as well as **plenty of mineral-and fiber-rich foods, like whole grains and fresh vegetables.**

- **Water** - During menopause, it is also important for women to get **plenty of water.** "One of the best things you can do during this time is to be sure **to drink plenty of quality water** -- at least **2 quarts daily or 1.9 litres or 8 to 9 cups**," writes Phyllis A. Balch, author of "Prescription for Dietary Wellness."

---

70 http://www.naturalnews.com/019538_hot_flashes_womens_health.html#ixzz3sceGg0PA

"Drinking water replaces fluids lost to perspiration during hot flashes and can even prevent or minimize the hot flashes themselves."[71]

Foods to Avoid:

Eating a diet high in **white sugar, white bread, pasta, or any foods that are highly refined and/or processed**, will induce more hot flashes. Women should also stay away from such things like **cheeses, and decaffeinated drinks, chocolate, red wine and foods that are deep-fried or overly spicy.** They are typical hot flash triggers for many women

71 IBID

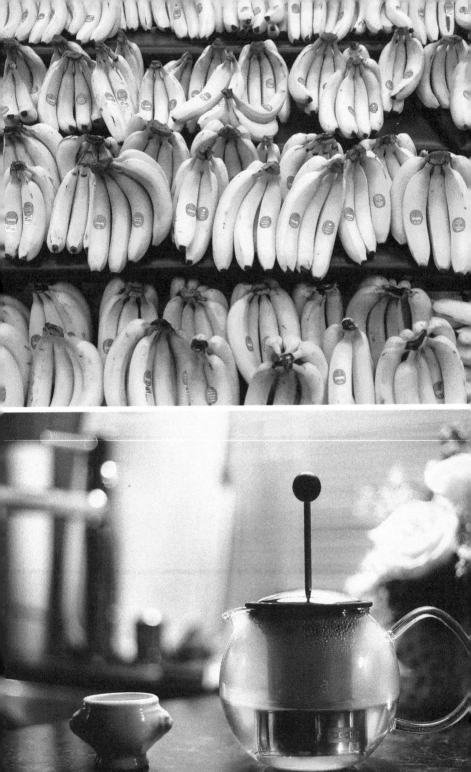

INSOMNIA[72]

Foods that Help One Sleep Better

- **Walnuts** - Walnuts are packed full of heart-healthy omega 3 fatty acids. They're also great for quality sleep. Walnuts are a good source of **tryptophan**, a sleep-enhancing amino acid that helps make **serotonin** and **melatonin**, the "body clock" hormone that sets your sleep-wake cycles. Melatonin is produced in the body by the pineal gland, and although the actual mechanism isn't all that well understood, it is commonly linked to improved sleep quality and regularity.

- **Bananas** - Bananas are one of the more well known sleep aiding foods. They are well-known for being rich in potassium, are also a good source of Vitamin

---

72 https://eunatural.
com/10-top-foods-to-eat-and-avoid-for-insomnia

B6, which is needed to make melatonin (a sleep-inducing hormone triggered by darkness), according to an article published in the *Annals of the New York Academy of Sciences.*[73]

- **Salad Leaves** - A freshly prepared salad is one of the best food choices you can make for good health. Romaine, chard, rocket and the like are all free from cholesterol, low in fat, and packed full of health promoting micronutrients. Those green leaves may also be one of the best choices you can make for your sleep.

Writer Diana Herrington explains:

The white fluid that you see when you break or cut lettuce leaves is called lactucarium. This has relaxing and sleep inducing properties like opium but without the strong side effects. Simply eat a few leaves or drink some lettuce juice.

Lettuce leaves are also rich in protein, and can have an alkalizing effect on the body, bringing down inflammation and reducing the risk of certain diseases

- **Tart Cherry Juice** -In a small study, melatonin-rich tart cherry juice was shown to aid sleep. When adults with chronic insomnia drank a cup of tart cherry juice twice a day they experienced some relief

---

73 http://www.eatingwell.com/nutrition_health/
nutrition_news_information/9_foods_to_help_you_sleep

in the severity of their insomnia[74]. A 2010 study also showed that "when compared to placebo, the study beverage produced significant reductions in insomnia severity".[75]

- **Cherries**, particularly (the tart variety), are a natural source of tryptophan and melatonin, which as mentioned above, are both involved with regulating sleep.

They also contain proanthocyanins, pigments that reduce inflammation and decrease the breakdown of tryptophan, allowing it to work for longer in the body.

The juice may also spike blood sugar levels slightly. This prompts the body to increase the production of insulin, which encourages the body towards a sleepier state.

- **Sweet Potatoes** - Sweet potatoes, a key ingredient in the diet of the Okinawans, who are some of the healthiest and longest living people on the planet. They are rich in Vitamin A, helping to improve ocular health and boost the immune system. Aside from being a health promoting superfood, sweet potatoes can also help to combat sleep deprivation. They are another great source of potassium, the micronutrient that encourages muscles to relax. Sweet

---

74   IBID

75   https://eunatural.
     com/10-top-foods-to-eat-and-avoid-for-insomnia

potatoes also contain Vitamin B6, and a dose of sleep inducing complex carbohydrates.

- **Kale** - This cruciferous vegetable is packed full of protein and health promoting micronutrients, most notably calcium. As well as promoting strong bones, calcium helps the brain to convert tryptophan to melatonin, essential for a good night's sleep.

- **Herbal tea** - Herbal teas are another useful remedy for insomnia. They can help you to distress and develop a sense of calm. Chamomile is one of the most popular when it comes to its sedative effect. As well as being a relaxant, it also has anti-inflammatory properties that can help with any joint aches and back pain, which may encourage you to a more restful state.

- **Chickpeas** - Chickpeas are one of the more surprising sleep aids. They're a great source of tryptophan, as well as containing a healthy dose of Vitamin B6, the same sleep promoting micronutrient found in bananas. They also contain calcium, which as mentioned above, helps the brain convert tryptophan to melatonin.

- **Wild Game** - Wild game meats such as elk and deer are packed full of protein needed to repair muscle tissue and stimulate growth. They are also lower in fat than other red meats, and often higher in health promoting micronutrients. Game meats commonly contain high levels of tryptophan, that same amino acid that keeps popping up, needed for the syntheses of important sleep hormones.

- **Grapefruit** - Grapefruit is packed full of Vitamin C, needed to maintain a healthy immune system. It's also a great source of sleep-friendly B-Vitamins and dietary fibre. Grapefruit is also a potent source of lycopene, a pigment that has been linked to healthier sleeping patterns.

The Foods to Avoid

Fast food – Avoid foods such as **burgers, fries, pizzas and kebabs** which are often packed full of disease promoting saturated fats and salts, whilst being void of any nutritional value.

The high fat content of many of these convenience foods stimulate the production of stomach acid. Sometimes this can overflow into the oesophagus, leading to heartburn, which can keep you awake for some time.

The high salt content of these foods dehydrates the body, which can lead to interrupted sleep.

Fast foods are often difficult to digest, which can inhibit the production of the sleep hormone melatonin.

Alcohol - Although drinking alcohol may seem like a good way to relax and de-stress, it probably does you more harm than good. It is better to swap a glass of wine (or two) in the evening with something more sleep friendly like chamomile tea.

Coffee & Tea

Caffeine is the other common remedy to an exhausting day at the office. Unfortunately, too much caffeine can significantly reduce the quality of your sleep. Caffeine has a half-life of around five hours (meaning it takes five hours for half of the caffeine to dissipate) so it may be wise to avoid drinking any coffee or other caffeinated drinks after lunch, and opt for water or herbal teas instead.

Energy Drinks - Energy drinks are packed full of caffeine, which as mentioned above, will not help your sleep quality. Many of the energy drinks are **high in sugar** and full of **artificial ingredients**. Plain old water or herbal teas are better for you.

A Large Evening Meal - It can be tempting to eat a big meal for dinner, especially if you have been exercising or had a busy day in the office. But as wellness advocate, Joy Bauer explains: "Eating a huge dinner, or even a large before-bedtime snack, may make you feel drowsy, but the sleep won't necessarily take. When you lie down and try to sleep, there's a good chance you'll feel uncomfortably full, which can keep you awake. Even worse, you may develop heartburn or gas, which will only increase your discomfort."[76] Instead of a large meal at dinner, try to make sure you are getting enough health promoting food in throughout the day, and go for a lighter evening meal whenever possible.

Pork and Cheese - Both pork and cheese are high in fat and can sometimes be difficult for the body to digest. This can make it harder for the body to utilise serotonin, hampering your ability to sleep deeply. According to health writer Melanie Haiken, they also contain the amino acid tyramine, which the body converts into noradrenalin. Noradrenalin is a stress hormone that raises the blood pressure and helps put the body into the 'fight or flight mode' – useful if there is an approaching wild predator, but not so great if you are trying to sleep.[77]

---

76 http://www.joybauer.com/insomnia/how-food-affects-sleep.aspx

77 http://www.health-conscious-travel.com/2009/09/21/
    hate-insomnia-5-foods-that-sabotage-sleep/

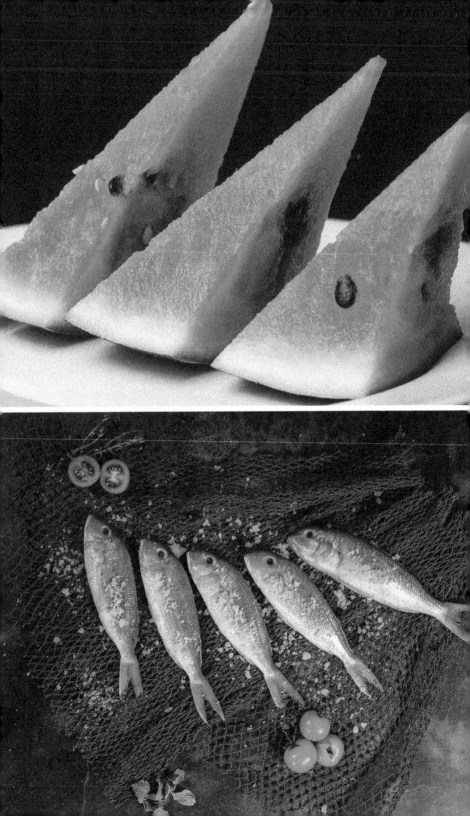

MIGRAINE

Foods to Relieve Migraines

- **Water** is a nutrient, essential for your body's proper functioning, and dehydration is a common migraine trigger. Migraine sufferers need to try and pre-empt thirst. Drink at least nine cups of liquid a day for women and 13 cups a day for men is recommended by most health experts. Water is the single best way to stay hydrated, but **herbal tea, decaf coffee, and fat-free or 1 percent reduced-fat milk** are also good choices. **Soda, sugary fruit drinks, sweetened tea or coffee, and juices should be avoided because they're too high in calories and sugar (and in some instances, are migraine triggers).**[78]

---

78 http://www.womansday.com/food-recipes/advice/g2387/
    foods-help-headache

- **Magnesium** may protect your body from the effects of a headache by relaxing blood vessels. Migraine sufferers may also experience relief by following a diet rich in magnesium, some experts believe. Try consuming magnesium-rich foods such as **bananas, dried apricots, avocados, almonds, legumes, cashews, brown rice** and other **whole grains, such as sorghum and millet.** Other foods best for magnesium also include s**pinach, sweet potatoes, white potatoes, Swiss chard, fresh amaranth, quinoa, sunflower seeds.**

- **Calcium** – Calcium rich foods also help to abate migraines. Foods such as plain, fat-**free yoghurt, leafy-greens and seeds.**[79]

- **Healthy Fats** - Adding certain kinds of fats into your diet may help reduce inflammation, which is thought to exacerbate migraine pain. Omega-3 fatty acids, which are mostly concentrated in **fatty fish**, and the monounsaturated fats found in **olive oil** have both been shown to reduce the frequency, duration, and severity of headaches.

- **Riboflavin** - Riboflavin — also called **vitamin B2** — is necessary for the body's production of energy at the level of the cell. Some research suggests that people with migraines may have a genetic defect that makes

---

79 IBID

it difficult for their cells to maintain energy reserves, and this lack of basic energy could trigger migraines. Although it is difficult to get enough riboflavin to prevent migraines from food sources alone, adding some riboflavin-rich foods to your diet will help. Good choices are **lean beef, a bowl of whole-grain fortified cereal with fat-free or reduced-fat milk, mushrooms, broccoli, and spinach.**

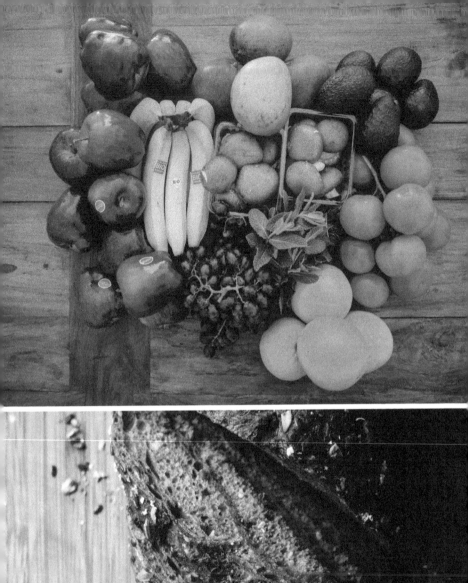
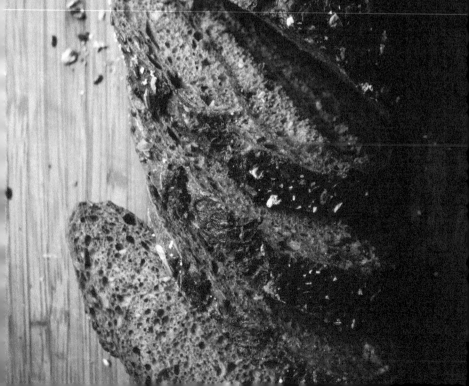

OBESITY

Foods to Lose Weight

Eat Well - Calories matter for weight and some foods make it easier for us to keep our calories in check. Healthy eating is a key to good health as well as maintaining a healthy weight. It is not only what and how much we eat but also, it seems, how we eat that is important.[80]

What to Eat - Choose minimally processed, whole foods, mostly plant based

- Add **Apple Cider Vinegar** to your vegetable salad. This helps to curb your appetite, potentially leading to greater weight loss. One 12-week study in obese individuals also showed that 15 or 30 ml of vinegar per day caused weight loss of 2.6–3.7 pounds, or

---

80 https://www.hsph.harvard.edu/obesity-prevention-source/
    diet-lifestyle-to-prevent-obesity/

1.2–1.7 kilograms[81] I add one tablespoon of Apple Cider Vinegar and or one tablespoon of lemon juice to a glass of warm water everyday and drink for cleansing and weight loss. (Use straw as lemon and Apple Cider Vinegar can ruin your teeth).

· **Whole grains (whole wheat, steel cut oats, brown rice, quinoa, sorghum, millet)**

· **Vegetables (a colorful variety)**:

  Leafy greens are an excellent addition to your weight loss diet. Not only are they low in calories but also high in fiber that helps keep you feeling full.

  Cruciferous vegetables which include **broccoli, cauliflower, cabbage and Brussels sprouts** are low in calories but high in fiber and nutrients. Adding them to your diet is not only an excellent weight loss strategy but may also improve your overall health.

· **Fish, especially Salmon** is high in both protein and omega-3 fatty acids, making it a good choice for a healthy weight loss diet. It is also very satisfying, keeping you full for many hours with relatively few calories. **Tuna** is an excellent, lean source of high-quality protein. Replacing other macronutrients, such as carbs or fat, with protein is an effective weight loss strategy on a calorie-restricted diet.

81 https://www.healthline.com/ nutrition/20-most-weight-loss-friendly-foods#section12

- **Boiled potatoes** are among the most filling foods. They're particularly good at reducing your appetite, potentially suppressing your food intake later in the day.

- Eating **unprocessed lean meat (beef or poultry)** is an excellent way to increase your protein intake. Replacing some of the carbs or fat in your diet with protein could make it easier for you to lose excess fat.

- **Beans and legumes** are a good addition to your weight loss diet. They're both high in protein and fiber, contributing to feelings of fullness and a lower calorie intake

- **Nuts, seeds and other healthful sources of protein**

- **Whole fruits (not fruit juices)**

  Avocados are a good example of a healthy fat source you can include in your diet while trying to lose weight. Just make sure to keep your intake moderate.

- Eating **lean dairy products, such as cottage cheese,** is one of the best ways to get more protein without significantly increasing your calorie intake.

- **Plant oils (olive and other vegetable oils)**

- **Drink water or other beverages that are naturally calorie-free.**

Tropical Foods

- **Okra** Okra's dietary fiber helps you feel full for longer, which will keep you from snacking on stray junk foods after Dinner.

- **Black jack leaves** have a lot of fiber which minimizes belly fat, the most dangerous form of fat to carry. Belly fat, also referred to as visceral fat, surrounds vital organs like the heart and liver and so this can prevent cardiovascular problems

How to Eat – Take time to chew and enjoy your food and have planned meal and snack times instead of mindless eating.

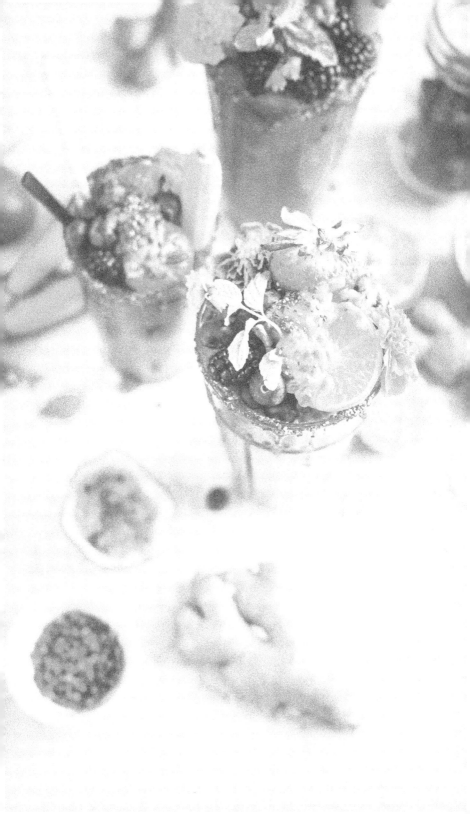

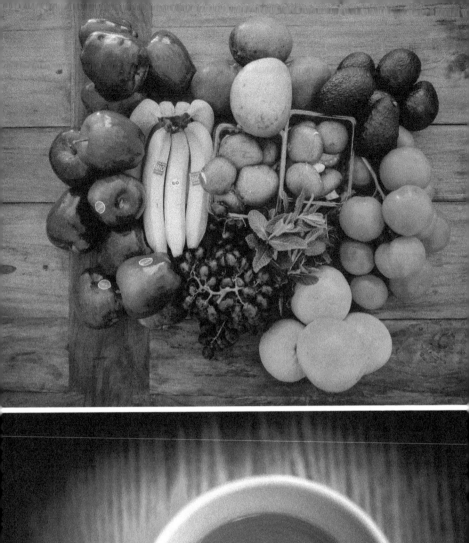
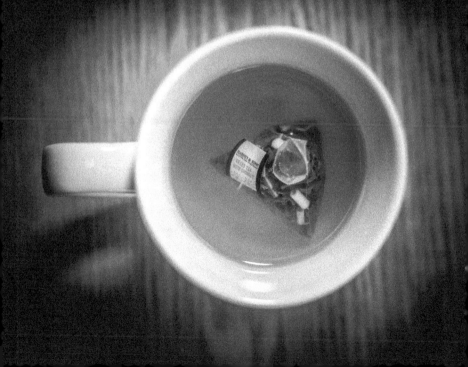

ODOUR – BAD BODY OR BREATH
Foods to Help With Bad Odour

- **Fiber-laden Foods** – To avoid body odor, avoid processed foods and eat more of plant-based foods, such as **fresh vegetables, legumes and fruits**. Plant foods contain fiber, which helps clean you out by maintaining regular digestion. A green salad with baby **kale and spinach** that includes lots of other raw vegetables -- including **carrots, peppers and cucumber** at most meals helps increase your intake of plant foods. Avoid eating too much broccoli, cauliflower and cabbage, as the sulfur in this brassica genus can cause body odor. **Citrus fruits** are another way to add fiber to your diet, and the acid in them readily flushes through your body, dismissing compounds that could cause lingering odor. Have **grapefruit** for breakfast or have an **orange** as a snack.

- **Herbs**- Seasoning foods with garlic and onion frequently, can make your body smell like these foods. Herbs that contain large amounts of chlorophyll, the compound that makes leaves green, can counteract body odor. **Wheatgrass juice** and herbs such as **parsley, cilantro and mint**, are examples of these foods. Drink wheatgrass straight and mix the herbs into steamed vegetables, salad dressings and pesto.

- **Gut Health** - Consume **probiotic-rich foods** to help restore good intestinal bacteria and to aid your digestion so that it processes foods more smoothly, and with less odor. **Fermented tea, known as kombucha, yogurt, fresh sauerkraut and pickles, Korean kimchi and kefir** are good choices for this.[82]

---

82 http://www.livestrong.com/
    article/155243-foods-to-eliminate-body-odor/

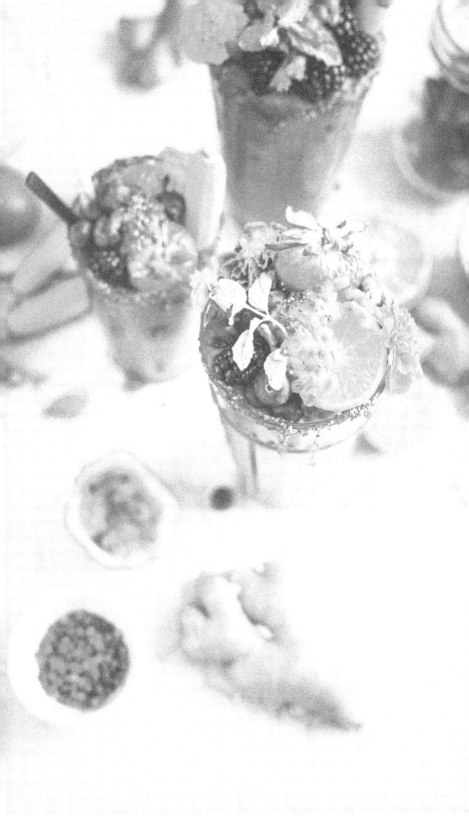

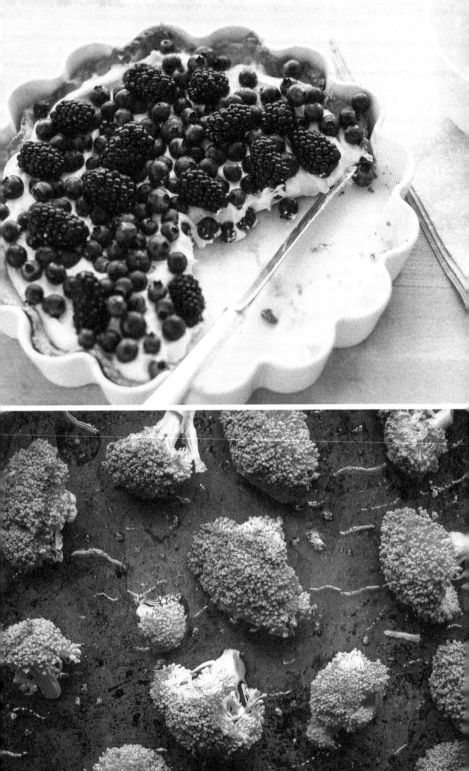

SEXUAL LIBIDO

Foods to enhance or boost Libido [83]

- **Black Raspberries** - Both the berries and the seeds will help you feel like it. Eat a handful a day and avoid any bedroom boredom. "This phytochemical-rich food enhances both libido and sexual endurance..."[84] Consume 10 black raspberries or a tablespoon of seeds a few hours before the game begins.

- **Broccoli** - The Vitamin C in this vegetable aids in blood circulation to organs and has also been associated with an improved female libido.

---

83 http://www.fitnessmagazine.com/mind-body/sex/
libido-boosting-foods/

84 Drs. Anna Maria and Brian Clement, authors of 7 Keys to Lifelong
Sexual Vitality and directors of Hippocrates Health Institute in
West Palm Beach, Florida.

- **Cloves** - This sex superfood is versatile when it comes to cooking: It can be brewed in hot apple cider, infused in your favorite exotic dish, or added to a chai tea latte. It helps both males and females. "In India, cloves have been used to treat male sexual dysfunction for centuries," says Glassman. Research published in the journal *BMC Complementary and Alternative Medicine* agrees, discovering that clove extracts produced an increase in the sexual activity of normal male rats.

- **Watermelon** - This is a sweet libido-booster. Although it is 92 percent water, that remaining 8 percent of fruit is jam-packed with vital nutrients for sexual health. Researchers at the Texas A&M Fruit and Vegetable Improvement Center reported finding in 2008 that watermelon has ingredients that delivered Viagra-like effects to the human body's blood vessels and could even aid in increasing libido. "Watermelon contains a phytonutrient called citrulline, which the body converts to arginine, an amino acid that boosts nitric oxide levels in the body, which relax blood vessels in the same way a medicine like Viagra does," say Drs. Clement.

- **Eggs** - A couple of eggs will make you feel refreshed and ready. "Eggs are high in protein, which is a source of stamina, and they're also low in calories," Glassman says. "In addition, they're a good source for an amino acid L-arginine, which has been shown to be effective in treating types of heart ailments and erectile dysfunction."

- **Ginseng** - Researchers at the University of Hawaii found that women who took a ginseng supplement significantly upped their libido in a month, and 68 percent also said their overall sex life improved dramatically. Add ginseng into your diet or try one of the many ginseng teas available.

- **Lettuce** - A small salad with oil and vinegar as dressing will help your waistline and rev your sex drive. "Iceberg lettuce contains an opiate that helps to activate sex hormones," say Drs. Clement and Nosh.

- **Ginger** - "King Henry VII and the ancient Asians were astute when using ginger for medicinal purposes," say Drs. Clement. "In the 21st century, those of us who know about botanical-ceuticals know that ginger helps circulation temperature adjustment, mucoid detoxification (mucus-like residue that can coat your GI tract) and a libido enhancer." Whether raw, in supplement form, or added to your favorite recipe or drink, ginger also lends itself to defense against winter's hard cold and flu season.

Other Foods that Help

Asparagus, Avocados, Chilies, Chocolate, Lemons, Nuts, Olives, Honey, Saffron

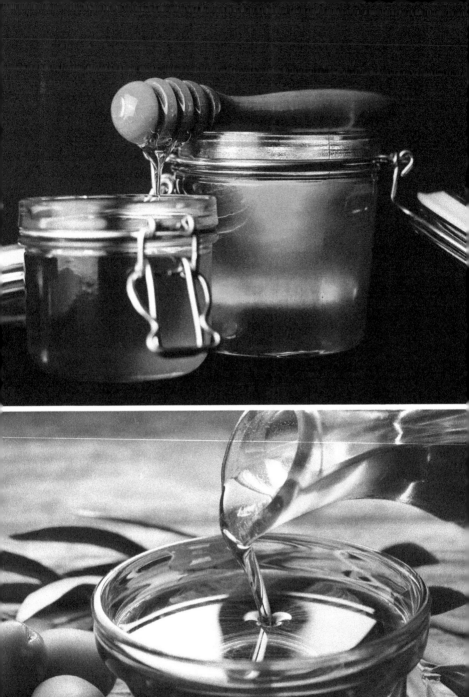

SNORING[85]

Foods to Soften Snoring

Snoring is a common affliction in modern society. Snoring can disrupt sleep, annoy sleep partners and might pose serious health consequences. To control your problem and have peaceful sleep for good, try the following foods:

- **Soy Milk** – Cows' milk can promote snoring, especially in those who have lactose sensitivities. The problem results from the special proteins in cow's milk that can cause serious allergic reactions. The allergic reactions enhance the congestion that will close the nasal passage and lead to snoring. Most doctors suggest that snorers should not drink cows' milk for preventing making their condition worse. Instead of consuming cow milk, you should drink soy milk which is a great alternative.

---

85 http://vkool.com/foods-and-tips-to-stop-snoring

- **Honey** - Honey is an anti-inflammatory as well as an anti-microbial. Consume honey to reduce the swelling in your throat which is the cause of snoring. It is best if you can add honey to tea before going to bed each night. This tip is applied by many well-known opera singers in the world to relax their throat and decrease crowding around the larynx as well. Thus, it can work successfully for us. Using honey, you can reduce snoring by decreasing crowding in the throat from the soft palate to the larynx.

- **Eat Fish and Avoid Red Meat** - This sounds to be controversial; however, there is a link between meat and snoring. Meat is inflammatory as it contains saturated fat causing slight spasms in the arteries. Therefore, it is necessary for you to cut down the portion of red and greasy meats for one or two weeks to see whether it is useful for you. In other words, you must be amazed that fish can be taken as snoring solution. It seems strange but it is reality. Intake white meat and fish is recommended for snorers. When it comes to fish for snoring, you should eat **tuna blue fish** due to its amazing effectiveness to snoring condition.

- **A Low-Carb Diet** - This kind of diet can assist you in reducing snoring by restoring your insulin balance. The reason is that sleep arena is a component of the insulin resistance syndrome; thus, if you consume a low-carb diet, you can improve the sleep arena significantly.

- **Tea** - The connection between tea and snoring is proven strongly. Some hot teas can help people lessen their snoring. Tea reduces congestion and phlegm. Chamomile coming with honey and lemon, common black tea with honey and lemon, white tea, and green tea are associated with the reduction of congestion. Thus, you can add tea into the daily diet to take control of your snoring condition naturally.

- **Eat Onions** - Onions are not only anti-inflammatory but also antioxidants. They also serve as decongestants that can clear the passage for air to pass through and thereby preventing snoring. Include onions in your daily diet to see what they can do for your problem.

- **Olive Oil** - It is good if you choose olive oil rather than saturated fat like butter. Saturated oil can result in forming acid reflux which may lead to heartburn if it remains confined to the stomach. In contrary, olive oil acts as anti-inflammatory and decrease arterial inflammation.

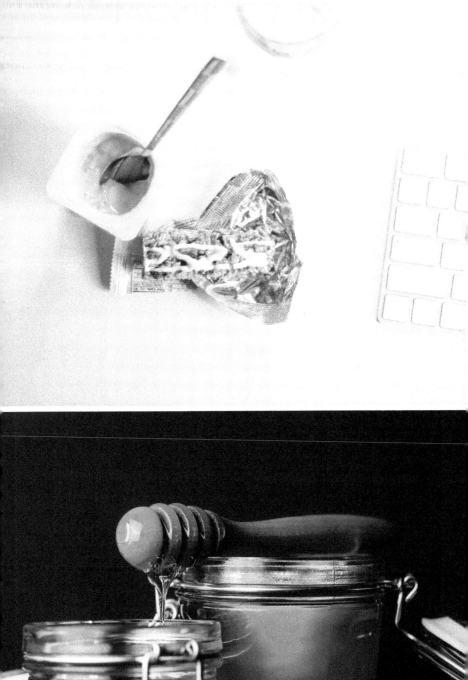

ULCERS[86]

Foods That Can Heal Ulcers

- **Honey**: Because honey fights bacteria, hospitals and clinics sometimes apply it to burns and other open wounds. These healing reasons can help heal an ulcer.

- **Broccoli, Brussels Sprouts, Cauliflower, and Kale**: These cruciferous vegetables all contain sulforaphane, a compound that appears to squelch H. pylori. In one study, after patients who tested positive for the bacteria ate a half cup of broccoli sprouts twice daily for seven days, 78 percent tested negative for the bacteria.

- **Cabbage**: The amino acid glutamine gives cabbage its anti-ulcer punch. Glutamine helps to fortify the mucosal lining of the gut and to improve blood flow

---

86 http://www.healthfitnessrevolution.com/foods-fight-ulcers/

to the stomach. This means it not only helps prevent ulcers but can also speed healing of existing sores.

- **Green Tea:** Has healing properties in the whole body, including the stomach, esophagus, and duodenum[87].

- Foods like **yogurt and kefir** (fermented milk) contain "good" bacteria that can inhibit H. pylori and may help ulcers heal faster. In one large study in Sweden, people who ate fermented milk products like yogurt at least three times a week were much less likely to have ulcers than people who ate yogurt less often.

- **Unripe Plantain**: This large, green, banana-like fruit is starchy and sticky in texture. It helps to soothe inflamed and irritated mucous membranes and has some antibacterial properties on top. Studies on rats with ulcers caused by daily aspirin use have shown that unripe green plantain can both prevent the formation of ulcers and help to heal them.

- **Foods High in Fiber:** Besides keeping you regular, fibre has a role in keeping ulcers at bay, especially those in the duodenum. Several studies have found that people who eat high-fiber diets have a lower risk of developing ulcers.

---

87 http://healthfitnessrevolution.
   com/10-good-reasons-to-drink-green-tea/

Foods to Avoid

Drinks that increase acid production can worsen an existing ulcer and cause more pain by also irritating your stomach lining.

Foods that might increase acid production include **alcohol, coffee** — including decaffeinated coffee — **carbonated beverages and fruit juices with citric acid.**

Milk, once the mainstay of ulcer diets, is now considered to increase acid production and worsen ulcers, although it might have a temporary soothing effect.[88]

88 IBID

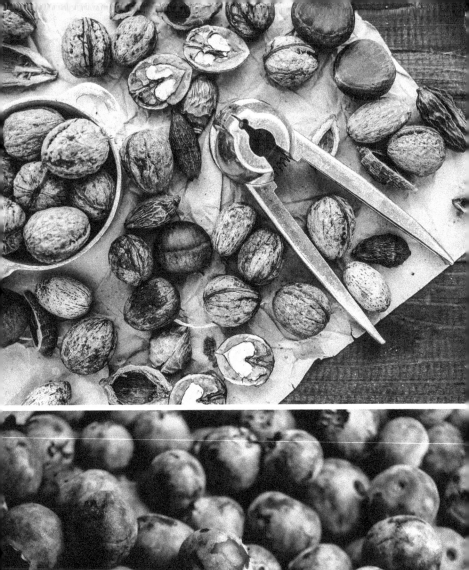
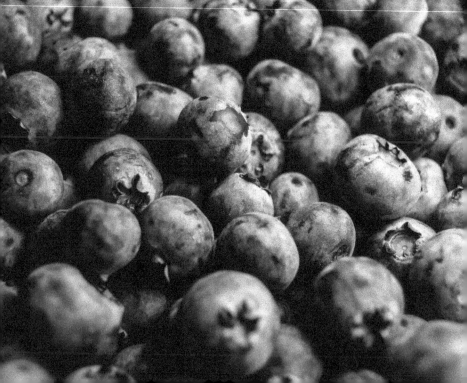

Other Tips for Good Health

I would like to add some facts on breaking a fast as I have seen this becoming a big problem to a lot of religious people who fast and fail to break properly.

FOODS FOR BREAKING A FAST[89]

Care needs to be taken when breaking a fast so as not to overburden your digestive system. The best benefit of fasting is realized when a fast is broken properly. Taking it slow and easy is not only kind to your body, but allows you the opportunity to integrate your new-found clarity on your relationship to food.

During a fast, the body undergoes several biological changes. Enzymes normally produced by the digestive

---

89   http://www.allaboutfasting.com/breaking-a-fast.html

system have ceased to be produced or have been diminished greatly, depending on the type of fast performed, so introducing food slowly allows the body time to re-establish this enzyme production.

The protective mucus lining of the stomach may be temporarily diminished as well, making the stomach walls more vulnerable to irritation until it also returns to normal. Gentle reintroduction of foods, beginning with the simplest and easiest-to-digest foods, supports this process. Substances known to be irritating to the system, such as coffee and spicy foods, must be avoided during the breaking process.

Because of these biological changes, overeating immediately following a fast is much worse than overeating at any other time. Your system needs time to readjust back to normal digestion and assimilation. Not taking the proper measures can result in stomach cramping, nausea, and even vomiting.

The adjustment period necessary is based on the length of the fast. Four days is considered adequate for any of the longer fasts, 1-3 days for shorter fasts, and just a day or so for one-day fasts.

Foods to use for breaking a fast

The most nutritious and easy-to-digest foods are used to break a fast initially, gradually adding more diversity and complexity over time.

The type of fast employed will determine the type of foods you use to break it. While juice or fruit are good for breaking a <u>water fast</u>, obviously, they aren't very helpful in breaking <u>juice</u> or <u>fruit fasts</u>.

To help you determine when to introduce the different food groups, use the following list. It begins with those that are easiest on the system and can be introduced early on, and progresses to those that should be added later.

Depending on the length of your fast, you may go through the list in one day or in 4 days. And you certainly don't need to eat everything on the list, it's just a general guideline.

- **fruit and vegetable juices**
- **raw fruits**
- **vegetable or bone broths**
- **yogurt (or other living, cultured milk products), unsweetened**
- **lettuces and spinach (can use plain yogurt as a dressing and top with fresh fruit)**
- **cooked vegetables and vegetable soups**

- raw vegetables
- well cooked grains and beans
- nuts and eggs
- milk products (non-cultured)
- meats and anything else

Any of the first three items are good for that initial "breaking" of a fast, that first thing you eat; raw fruit being the easiest and most popular.

Even if you did a brown rice fast, eating at #8 on the list, you'll want to start adding new foods from toward the top of the list. This will support re-establishment of more diverse enzyme production beginning with the simplest.

More pointers for breaking a fast

Pay close attention to your body's reactions to these "new" foods. Watch for any adverse reactions, perhaps signalling a mild allergy or that you have gone too far, too quickly. Feel for the sensation of fullness and stop eating at that point. Begin to train yourself to watch for that signal, so you'll always know when your body is fully nourished.

When breaking a fast, begin with frequent small meals, every 2 hours or so, progressing gradually toward larger meals with more time in between them until you reach a "normal" eating routine, such as 3 meals and 2 snacks in a day's time.

Chew foods well. This will help immensely with proper digestion and is a good habit to foster.

Strive to add live enzymes and good bacteria to your system. Fresh, raw foods are full of living enzymes good for your body and digestion. Probiotics, or "good" bacteria, can be found not only in pill form, but also in naturally cultured and fermented food products, such as yogurt, sauerkraut, and miso.

Overall, the following four factors represent what we are trying to accomplish when breaking a fast:

Frequent meals --- toward less frequent meals

Small meals --- toward larger meals

Easy to digest --- toward harder, requiring more enzymes, to digest

Less variety --- toward more variety

While it may take a little thought and attention, breaking a fast properly is so important to our overall health and to reaping the full benefits fasting can create.[90]

---

[90] IBD

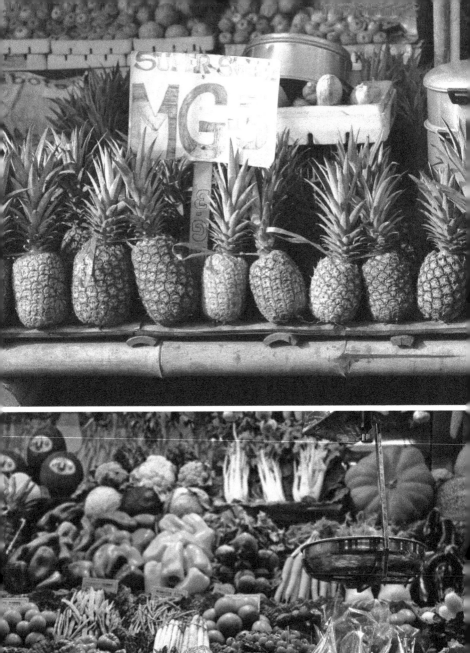
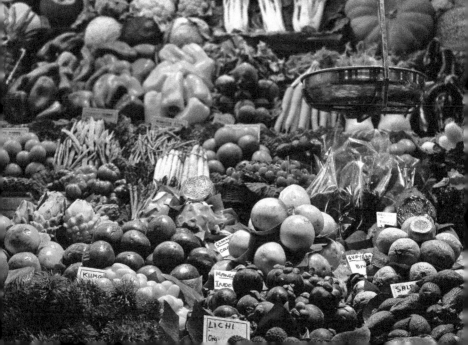

Other Important Factors to Good Health

In addition to eating the right foods, one needs to observe the following:

PHYSICAL ACTIVITY

As a general goal, aim for at least 30 minutes of physical activity every day. If you want to lose weight or meet specific fitness goals, you may need to exercise more. Want to aim even higher? You can achieve more health benefits, including increased weight loss, if you exercise up to 300 minutes a week.[91]

---

91   http://www.mayoclinic.org/healthy-lifestyle/fitness/
     expert-answers/exercise/faq

DRINK PLENTY OF WATER

So how much fluid does the average, healthy adult living in a temperate climate need? The Institute of Medicine determined that an adequate intake (AI) for men is roughly about 13 cups (3 liters) of total beverages a day. The AI for women is about 9 cups (2.2 liters) of total beverages a day.

Everyone has heard the advice, "Drink eight 8-ounce glasses of water a day." That's about 1.9 liters, which isn't that different from the Institute of Medicine recommendations. Although the "8 by 8" rule isn't supported by hard evidence, it remains popular because it's easy to remember. Just keep in mind that the rule should be reframed as: "Drink eight 8-ounce glasses of fluid a day," because all fluids count toward the daily total.[92]

I found the following article interesting and I have been following it and see the benefits:

JAPANESE WATER THERAPY[93]

According to Japanese tradition, water therapy can be used as a natural treatment for diabetes, gastritis, headache, asthma, bronchitis, arthritis, epilepsy, heart problems, tuberculosis, kidney and urine diseases, diarrhea,

---

92 IBD

93 http://www.healthyandnaturalworld.com/
what-happen-when-you-drink-water-on-an-empty-stomach/

vomiting, constipation, hemorrhoids, eye diseases, ear nose and throat diseases, problems with the uterus, cancer and menstrual disorders.

The practice should be performed first thing in the morning.

1. Before brushing your teeth, drink 640 ml (4 glasses of 160 ml) of water. Ideally, the water shouldn't contain fluoride.

2. Brush and clean your mouth, but don't eat or drink anything for another 45 minutes.

3. Have your breakfast as normal.

4. After breakfast, don't eat anything for 2 hours.

According to the original Japanese tradition, the water should be slightly warm, and not cold or room temperature. In the Far East, people usually don't drink cold water with their meals. Instead, warm tea is offered.

How Often You Should Drink Water on An Empty Stomach

According to the Japanese tradition, the practice of drinking water on an empty stomach should be done regularly and different time frames are predicted to treat, improve or control different conditions:

1. High blood pressure – 30 days

2. Diabetes – 30 days

3. Gastritis – 10 days

4. Constipation – 10 days

5. Tuberculosis – 90 days

6. Cancer – 180 days

7. People who suffer from arthritis should do the therapy for only three days in their first week, and then progress to a daily treatment.

It is suggested that if you initially struggle to drink such a large amount of fluids first thing in the morning, start with a smaller amount and then gradually increase to 4 glasses.

ENOUGH SLEEP

While sleep requirements vary slightly from person to person, most healthy adults need between 7 to 9 hours of sleep per night to function at their best. Children and teens need even more. And despite the notion that our sleep needs decrease with age, most older people still need at least 7 hours of sleep. Since <u>older adults often have trouble sleeping</u> this long at night, daytime naps can help fill in the gap.

The best way to figure out if you're meeting your sleep needs is to evaluate how you feel as you go about your day. If you're logging enough hours, you'll feel energetic and alert all day long, from the moment you wake up until your regular bedtime.

Foods to Avoid for best health

PROCESSED MEATS

This is a long list that includes, but is not limited to, sausages, hot dogs, bacon, most lunch meats like bologna or pimento loaf.

Researchers who wrote in the journal of BMC Medicine said that the excessive salts and chemicals that are used when making processed meats are damaging to your health. The study showed that 1 in every 17 people who were involved in the study died and those who ate 160 grams or more of processed meats increased their risk of early death as much as 44 percent within 12 years as opposed to those who ate 20 grams or less. This study involved people from 10 European countries and went on for almost 13 years.[94]

All these processed meats contain numerous chemicals and preservatives, including sodium nitrates, which make them, look appealing and fresh but are well known carcinogens. Smoking meats seem to be particularly bad as the meat picks up tar from the smoking process - the same deadly ingredient that cigarette smoke contains[95]

---

94 http://naturalon.com/10-of-the-most-cancer-causing-foods

95 IBID

MICROWAVE POPCORN

Those little bags of popcorn are so convenient but they are dangerous to your health. Conventional microwave popcorn bags are lined with a chemical called perfluorooctanoic acid (PFOA). This is a toxin you can find in Teflon also. According to a recent study at the University of California, PFOA is linked to infertility in women. Numerous studies in lab animals and humans show that exposure to PFOA significantly increases the risk of kidney, bladder, liver, pancreas and testicular cancers.

POTATO CHIPS

Potato chips are a cheap, great tasting, quick snack, however, the negative effects they have on your body may not be worth the little bit of pleasure you derive from these crispy snacks.

Potato chips are high in both fat and calories, which are sure to bring on weight gain. A study done in the New England Journal of medicine found that eating just 1 ounce of potato chips per day caused an average 2-pound weight gain in one year. Besides being full of trans-fats which can cause high cholesterol in most people, they have excessive sodium levels which, for many people, cause high blood pressure.

Potato chips have artificial flavors, numerous preservatives, and colors which are not good for you. Potato chips are fried in high temperatures to make them crispy but this also causes them to make a material called acrylamide, a known carcinogen that is also found in cigarettes.

As an alternative for the kids, buy them baked potato chips or tortilla chips which are at least lower in both fat and calories. Air popped popcorn and whole wheat pretzels are another healthier option. Or try baked apple chips or banana chips which are dehydrated. Both are crispy and are far healthier than regular potato chips.[96]

Hydrogenated oils

All hydrogenated oils are vegetable oils. Vegetable oils cannot be extracted naturally like butter but must be chemically removed from their source, and then they are changed to be more acceptable to consumers. They are frequently deodorized and colored to look appealing.

All vegetable oils contain high levels of Omega–6 fatty acids. An excess of Omega- 6 fatty acids causes health problems, such as heart disease and an increase in various cancers, especially skin cancer. You need a good balance of both Omega 3 and Omega 6. Try to get plenty of Omega 3 every day. You can do this in the form of supplements and grass fed meats. Also, fatty fish such as salmon and mackerel are a very good source of Omega 3.

Hydrogenated oils are used to preserve processed foods and keep them looking appealing Hydrogenated oils

96   IBID

influence our cell membranes' structure and flexibility, which is linked to cancer.

Foods that are highly salted, pickled, or smoked

Foods that are cured by use of nitrates or nitrites act as preservatives as well as adding color to the meat. Although nitrates do not cause cancer in and of themselves, under certain conditions these chemicals change once they are inside the body into N-nitroso composites. It's this N-nitroso that is associated with a greater increase in the risk of developing cancers.

Smoking foods such as meat or nuts causes these food items to absorb considerable amounts of the tar that smoke produces. Tar is a known carcinogen. Meats such as bacon, sausage, bologna, and salami are high in fat and salt. Pickled foods are also very high in salts.

There is overwhelming evidence that eating these types of foods greatly increases the risk of colorectal cancer and higher rates of stomach cancer. The rates of stomach cancer are much greater in places such as Japan where a traditional diet contains many foods that are highly salted, and/or smoked.

Highly processed white flours

Most of you have already heard by now that white flour is not a good thing, but you most likely have no idea just how bad it really is for your health. Refining grains destroys their natural nutrients. Mills now bleach flour with a chemical called chlorine gas.

The EPA states that chlorine gas is a dangerous irritant that is not safe to inhale and in large quantities can be lethal. White flour lurks in many processed foods. White processed flour has a very high glycemic rate which quickly raises the blood sugar level and insulin levels, which can be a direct cause of diabetes, not to mention it is believed that it spreads cancer cells by feeding the cells directly.

Cancerous tumors feed mostly on the sugars in your bloodstream. By avoiding refined grains such as white flour, you can avoid, or at the very least, starve tumors.[97]

REFINED SUGARS

Refined sugars are not only known to spike insulin levels, but also to be the most preferable food for cancer cells, thus promoting their growth.

Cancers seem to have a sweet tooth. This is a known fact that has been around for many years. The Nobel laureate in medicine, German Otto Warburg, back in 1931, first discovered that tumors and cancers both use sugars to "feed" themselves and/or to increase in size. To proliferate, cancer cells seem to prefer feeding on fructose-rich sweeteners like high-fructose corn syrup

---

[97] http://naturalon.com/10-of-the-most-cancer-causing-foods

(HFCS); the reason is that HFCS is being metabolized by cancer cells most quickly and easily.

Now it is clear why high-fructose corn syrup is considered the worst offender. And since cakes, pies, cookies, sodas, juices, sauces, cereals, and many other extremely popular, mostly processed, food items are loaded with refined sugars and HFCS in particular, this helps explain why cancer rates are on the rise these days.

Artificial Sweeteners

Most people use artificial sweeteners to either lose weight or because they are diabetic and must avoid sugar. The main problem in all this is that there are numerous studies that show people who consume artificial sweeteners on a regular basis, such as in sodas, or coffee sweeteners, gain weight. It also does little or nothing to help those with diabetes.

In fact, artificial sweeteners make it even more difficult to control their blood sugar levels and worsen conditions that are related to diabetes such as cataracts and gastroparesis. Sometimes aspartame has been found to cause convulsions, which some people will mistake for an insulin reaction.

Not to mention that artificial sweeteners inhibit your body's ability to monitor its daily calorie consumption and make the body crave even more sweets. Well, we've already discussed how refined sugars can cause cancer.

There is mounting evidence that the chemicals that make up these sweeteners, especially aspartame, break down in the body into a deadly toxin called DKP. When your stomach processes this chemical, it in turn produces chemicals that can cause cancer, especially brain tumors.[98]

DIET ANYTHING

Diet foods, including frozen foods, or prepackaged foods labeled as "diet" or "low fat", including diet sodas, generally contain aspartame, which is a chemical, artificial sweetener that we talk about in detail above. There are numerous studies showing that aspartame causes many diseases and sicknesses such as cancers, birth defects, and heart problems.

All "diet" food is chemically processed and made from super refined ingredients, excessive sodium levels, as well as artificial colors and flavors to make it taste good. Don't ever forget, artificial anything is NOT real food! Although the FDA says that all these added chemicals are safe to eat, you might want to take their advice with a grain of salt. After all, don't they also tell you that sugar and vegetable oils are safe to eat? (Not to mention GMO's and fast food!)

There have been many studies that show that these additives, for some people, can be addicting. They feed that "feel good" part in your brain, like cocaine!

98 IBID

ALCOHOL

An American study that followed the diet and lifestyles of more than 200,000 women for almost 14 years found that postmenopausal women who drank one drink per day or less had an almost 30 percent increase in breast cancer rates compared to women who did not drink at all.

In 2007, experts working for the World Health Organizations International Agency for Research on Cancer looked at the scientific evidence regarding cancer and alcohol use from 27 different studies. They found sufficient evidence to state the following: "Alcohol is a toxic substance related to more than 60 different disorders. For some chronic health conditions in which alcohol is implicated, such as breast cancer among women, there is an increasing risk with increasing levels of alcohol consumption, with no evidence of a threshold effect. For some other conditions, such as liver cirrhosis, the risk is curvilinear, increasing geometrically with increasing consumption"[99]

While a moderate or low consumption of alcohol can be healthy and lead to a reduced risk of heart disease, excessive drinking is known to cause heart failure, stroke, and sudden death. So an occasional glass of wine is not bad. The problem is excessive drinking of alcohol.

---

[99] http://www.who.int/substance_abuse/
expert_committee_alcohol_trs944

Red Meat

Evidence has shown that red meat in one's diet, in small, infrequent amounts is good for one. Grass fed beef contain conjugated linoleic acid that fights against certain cancers.

However, in a study done over a 10-year period, eating red meat every day, even a small amount increased a man's risk of dying from cancer by 22 percent and a woman's chance by 20 percent. A separate research study has shown that eating a lot of red meat increased the risk of breast, prostate, and colon cancer. **Red meat** seems particularly dangerous when talking about colon cancer. A study done in the US followed almost 150,000 people between the ages of 50 and 74. This study showed that the long-term consumption of red meat significantly increased the amount of colon cancer found in the subjects studied. On the other hand, the long-term consumption of fish and poultry appeared to be protective in nature.[100]

Tropical Foods for HEALTH AND HEALING

- **Black Jack** vegetable is known botanically as bidens pilosa and in South Africa local names include muxiji and gewone knapseherel. In Zimbabwe it is known as *tsine*. Like many indigenous African vegetables, black jack has an impressive nutritional profile that comes

---

100 http://naturalon.com/10-of-the-most-cancer-causing-foods

with a very wide variety of benefits. It is rich in fiber and antioxidants.

The antioxidants in black jack help keep the cardiovascular system in good health. Studies continue to show a strong relationship between diets rich in antioxidants and very low rates of cardiovascular diseases such as heart disease, high blood pressure, cholesterol abnormalities, and stroke. Other unprocessed plant foods also provide plenty of antioxidants.

The fiber and the antioxidants help in regulating blood sugar, which makes Black Jack great for prevention and treatment or Diabetes.

Black Jack also has powerful anti-cancer features.

- **OKRA** - Okra is a flowering plant that is known in many parts of the world as ladies fingers or bhindi.

DIABETES MANAGEMENT

Okra has potent antioxidant power in its seeds and peel, which specifically helps people with type 2 diabetes.

OKRA IMPROVES DIGESTION

The high amount of fiber in the vegetable helps improve the absorption process in the large intestine and stimulates peristalsis in the body. This also **helps prevent constipation.**

REDUCES FATIGUE

Research studies have suggested that okra consumption could be related to improved metabolic capacity and improved ability to manage stress as the vegetable results in less production of lactic acid which is related to fatigue.

- PUMPKIN LEAVES belong to the leafy vegetable family. These leaves are nutritious and are rich in vitamins and minerals

BENEFITS OF EATING PUMPKIN LEAVES

1. **Improves Eye Health**

Vitamin A present in pumpkin leaves helps in preventing degeneration of some of the parts of the eye, which otherwise would degrade with age. This can lead to a condition known as **Age-related Macula Degeneration** (ARMD).

2. **Lowers Cholesterol**

As there is a huge amount of fibre in these leaves, it reduces the absorption of bile acid and cholesterol, from the small intestines, thereby resulting in low levels of cholesterol and healthy heart!

3. **Increases Fertility** by curing any testicular damage and also by increasing the spermatogenesis

4. **Controls Diabetes** Pumpkin leaves are known to have the hypoglycaemic effect which helps in reducing

sugar levels in the blood, thus keeping diabetes under control!

5. **Antiageing** Due to the presence of anti-oxidants in abundance, these leaves are known to slow down the ageing process and to help in keeping bones and skin healthy.

6. **Cancer Prevention** The high amount of fibre, vitamins and minerals in pumpkin leaves help in cancer prevention

7. **Boosts Immunity** It helps in increasing haemoglobin in blood and in keeping bones strong. This decreases the risk of getting affected by diseases, thereby keeping you healthy.

8. The high fibre content **helps in digestion** and detoxification

9. Treats Anemia because of the rich content of iron and folate in these leaves

- **Pigweed** (Mowa in Shona) The plant is often considered to be an invasive weed, but like many weeds, it is quite edible and healthy to eat.

Benefits include:

1. Can be used as a laxative and improves overall health

2. With capsicum and onion, it can be used to **increase weight** and in a soup with garlic, tomato, pepper and cumin, it can be eaten **to lose weight.**

3. Pigweed contains omega 3 fatty acids and it helps in the brain development. It also prevents you from the symptoms of ADHD.

4. It purifies the blood and helps to recover the body from chronic illness. It increases the milk production in breast feeding mothers.

- SPIDER FLOWER LEAVES (Nyeve in Shona) plant has high levels of fiber, beta-carotene and Vitamin C. Many vegetables lose their Vitamin C when cooked but the spider flower retains the vitamins even after boiling it.

The vegetables have a significant amount of **Calcium, Magnesium and Iron minerals.** They also have a high supply of **Vitamin** A which is beneficial in improving eyesight

The high levels of antioxidants help to prevent diseases such as diabetes, cancer and heart diseases.

They are rich in protein and amino acids.

BENEFICIAL TO PREGNANT AND LACTATING WOMEN

The plant has been doing wonders when used in some communities to speed up the process of childbirth and ease labor pains. After giving birth, the women eat the vegetables to regain strength and improve lactation. It also helps to replenish lost blood after childbirth because of its rich iron content.

MEDICINAL VALUE

In some areas, the spider flower plant is used in the treatment of headaches, stomach aches, vomiting, constipation, Ear infection and diphtheria. Its anti-inflammatory properties can also be used to treat arthritis.

- COW PEAS (*nyemba* in **Shona**) are abundant and inexpensive but their nutritional value is far higher than most fancy foods. Due to its tolerance for sandy soil and low rainfall it is an important <u>crop</u> in the <u>semi-arid</u> regions across Africa and other countries.

Their health benefits includes improving digestion, supporting heart health, detoxifying the body, treating insomnia, managing diabetes, and supporting blood circulation. Other health benefits include preventing anemia, supporting weight loss, supporting healthy skin, fighting free radicals and maintaining healthier bones.

They can be added to stews, curries and also added to salads to add <u>protein</u> and carbohydrates.

- COW PEAS LEAVES are not only delicious when consumed but they also supply the body with numerous health benefits. According to James Duke in his Handbook of Legumes of World Economic Importance cow-pea leaves can produce 9 times the calories, 15 times the protein, 90 times the calcium, and thousands of times more vitamin

C and beta-carotene of cow-pea seed. [101] So the above benefits for the Cow Pea seeds are even more pronounced for the leaves.

- GUAVAS Leaves[102] - Fresh guava leaves contain antioxidants, antibacterial & anti-inflammatory properties and helpful tannins, therefore is considered as a natural pain reliever. The chemicals in guava leaves like carotenoids, polyphenols, flavonoids & tannins can be very effective in treating different diseases. Guava leaves

- lower blood sugar levels

- help boost heart health because of the higher levels of potassium and soluble fiber

- Relieve painful symptoms of menstruation

- Guavas are an excellent source of dietary fiber. Therefore, eating more guavas may aid healthy bowel movements and prevent constipation

- **Guavas help in weight loss:** With only 37 calories in one fruit and 12% of your recommended daily fiber intake, they are a filling, low-calorie snack

- **They boost immunity because of the high levels of Vitamin C in them**

---

101   https://www.malishobora.co.ke/
      kunde-or-cowpeas-is-an-all-rounder-vegetable/

102   https://www.sentinelassam.com/topheadlines/health-benefits-of-guava-one-of-the-most-underrated-fruit-494892

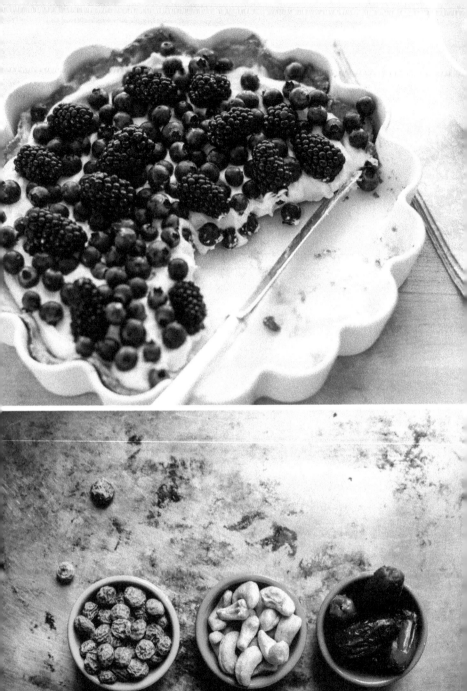
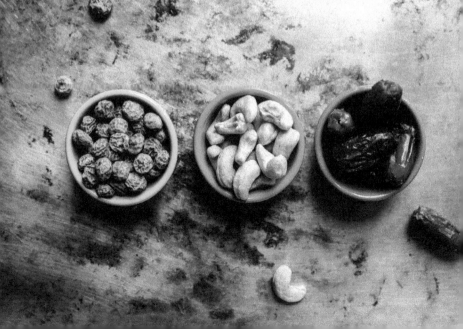

CONCLUSION

I hope that this book will help save someone from developing chronic ailments or other lifestyle problems. The contents in it have helped me and others a lot. In summary, the following foods keep occurring as good for a lot of problems:

Fruits, especially **berries**

Vegetables, especially broccoli and leafy greens

Whole grains

Fish, especially salmon

Olive Oil

Green Tea

Avocado

Nuts

Beans

These are also mostly in the Mediterranean diet, which makes it a great diet to follow.

CPSIA information can be obtained
at www.ICGtesting.com
Printed in the USA
BVHW090721160321
602631BV00001B/1